Tackling Mental Health Crises

Tackling Mental Health Crises

David Kingdon and Marie Finn

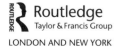
Routledge
Taylor & Francis Group

LONDON AND NEW YORK

First published 2006 by Routledge
27 Church Road, Hove, East Sussex BN3 2FA

Simultaneously published in the USA and Canada
by Routledge
270 Madison Avenue, New York, NY 10016

*Routledge is an imprint of the Taylor & Francis Group,
an informa business*

Typeset in Times by
RefineCatch Limited, Bungay, Suffolk
Printed and bound in Great Britain by
TJ International Ltd, Padstow, Cornwall
Paperback cover design by Terry Foley, Anú Design

This publication has been produced with paper manufactured to
strict environmental standards and with pulp derived from
sustainable forests.

British Library Cataloguing in Publication Data
A catalogue record for this book is available from the British Library

Library of Congress Cataloging-in-Publication Data
Kingdon, David G.
  Tackling mental health crises / David Kingdon & Marie Finn.
    p. ; cm.
  Includes bibliographical references and index.
  ISBN13: 978–1–58391–978–3 (hbk)
  ISBN10: 1–58391–978–3 (hbk)
  ISBN13: 978–1–58391–979–1 (pbk)
  ISBN10: 1–58391–979–1 (pbk)
    1. Crisis intervention (Mental health services)   2. Mental health
services.   I. Finn, Marie, 1964–   . II. Title.
    [DNLM: 1. Crisis Intervention–methods.   2. Mental Disorders–
therapy.   3. Mental Health Services.   WM 401 K54t 2006]
RC454.4.K532 2006
362.2′04251–dc22   2005035871

ISBN13: 978–1–58391–978–3 (hbk)
ISBN13: 978–1–58391–979–1 (pbk)

ISBN10: 1–58391–978–3 (hbk)
ISBN10: 1–58391–979–1 (pbk)

Contents

Introduction

Writing this book has been fascinating as we have explored the ways in which medical, psychological and social approaches can be integrated in tackling crises. We have learnt a great deal in researching it and hope you will find it useful in your work. It is aimed at mental health practitioners of all disciplines, especially those new to this work. But we also hope that those with experience working with adults will find something new in the approaches described here. Other professionals – family practitioners, generic social workers, general nurses and others – who encounter mental health crises may also find it useful.

A few introductory comments are needed. We have decided to use the term 'client' on the basis that it seems the most descriptive in the variety of circumstances that we discuss. Some people presenting in crisis do not have a health care problem so it would be inaccurate to call them 'patients' or 'users' of the services. Both these terms and others such as 'resident' may be more accurate in specific situations, or individuals might prefer them, but they could not be used consistently throughout the text. 'Client' also seems to have a tone of respect about it that we quite like. We have used 'carer' to mean someone giving care to others, although the term 'care-giver' from the USA has much to commend it. We hope the terms used do not interfere with your appreciation of the book.

Mental health legislation is referred to in the chapters on crisis planning and risk and we have taken the Council of Europe recommendation on psychiatry and human rights[1] as the basis for these discussions. However, we do refer to specific mental health legislation, for example, the Mental Health Act 1983 (applied in England and Wales) and the Scottish Act in certain areas where these Acts go further or are more detailed than the recommendation. But this is not intended to be a guide to the use of specific mental health legislation in crisis situations. While we give some general guidance, for example about where such use may need to be considered, we are assuming that those implementing involuntary measures will have been appropriately trained prior to being authorised to do so.

We have made the decision to be very selective with referencing as this is intended to be a handbook to learn about, and use in, crisis situations. The evidence base for most of the book is unfortunately very limited and so what we generally describe is based on our experience over the years. We have also consulted other books on crisis[2] and emergency psychiatry[3, 4] such as exist, and also clinical guidelines[5] where relevant. Where we think a suggestion may be controversial we have referenced it, if that is possible. We use end-notes for referencing to minimise disruption to the text.

We have discussed the use of medication frequently and tried to make this evidence-based while acknowledging varying practice. However, we have not attempted to provide comprehensive guidance on dosages, indications, contra-indications and side-effects, and the supplementary use of prescribing guides, of which there are many excellent texts,[6, 7] is commended.

Organising the book has taken some thought and has evolved as we have written it (see Figure 1). We have considered what sorts of crises clients may experience. We have taken a vulnerability–stress model acknowledging the social dimensions of crisis. We have then focused on symptoms and behaviour, for example, voices, anxiety, panic or self-harm, as opposed to psychiatric diagnostic categories as this seems the most inclusive, holistic and practical approach. (Psychiatric diagnosis is recognised as problematic and currently both of the internationally recognised systems are under review, at least in part, because of concerns about their validity and clinical utility.[8])

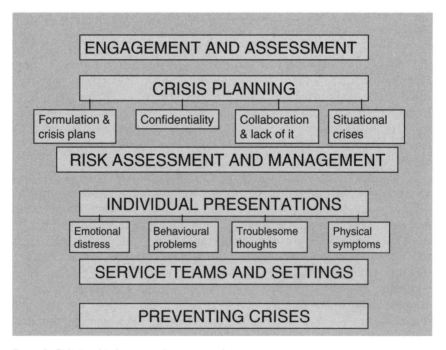

Figure 1 Relationship between diagnoses and symptoms

When somebody presents in crisis, it is usually the symptoms they are experiencing which present first ('I can't cope any more'), or in some circumstances it is the event bringing on the crisis that is initially presented ('My partner's left me'). Use of medication also fits with a symptomatic approach to a degree – we use anti-depressants when the person is depressed or anti-psychotic drugs when someone is presenting with psychotic symptoms. However, we also think in terms of psychiatric classifications at times (e.g. mania, schizophrenia, depressive illness, eating disorders or substance misuse), and this means that some cross-referencing will be needed between chapters and we have tried to assist with this wherever possible (see Figure 2).

We have started the book with general chapters about what a crisis is, including discussion of possible effects on staff members themselves, then the principles of assessment and engagement, moving on to planning interventions and handling risk and then looking at specific ways that clients present, i.e. with emotional distress, behavioural difficulties, troublesome thoughts and physical symptoms. Within each of these categories are a number of different presenting issues and Figure 3 illustrates this. It may be that clients will present with multiple presenting symptoms but generally there will be one that is most prominent and we have cross-referred to allow intervention with all. We have included case examples throughout and checklists as prompts for use in crisis situations.

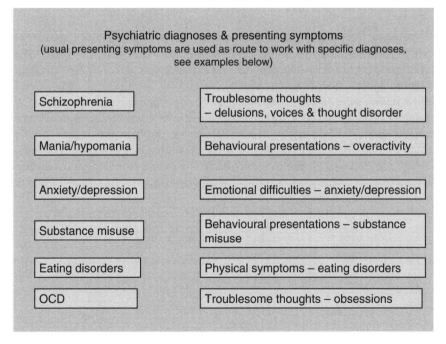

Figure 2 Chapter headings and individual symptoms

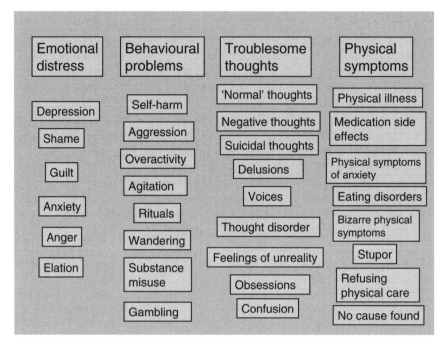

Figure 3 Organisation of book

The book then discusses the various service settings and teams that exist, in which crisis presentations occur and to which individuals can be referred. The book concludes with a chapter on preventing crises which is described in individual and societal terms.

Finally we would like to acknowledge the contribution made to our understanding of tackling crises by the many clients, carers and staff that we have worked with over the years in Bristol, Jersey, Nottinghamshire and especially Southampton. In particular, we would like to thank Jake, Bob, Dee, Carmel, Penny and Bedford House Self Harm Group whose comments giving their perspective on using services we have included, and also Jimmy and Carmel (thanks again) as carers.

Chapter 1

What is a crisis?

'Everything you ever feared in your life is put out on the table . . . you see things in different ways . . . you shouldn't be treated like that . . .'

Jake

When we talk about crises in the context of mental health services we are more often than not referring to episodes that are experienced by service users as being profoundly distressing. We can appreciate from the above statement what a harsh and bewildering experience a mental health crisis can be. In fact, mental health practitioners tend to use the word 'crisis' rather loosely, to include any time they are contacted by a client who is having a difficult time or who is facing a seemingly irresolvable difficulty. So we need to clarify what we really mean by a crisis.

In classic crisis intervention theory, a crisis is 'an upset in a steady state'[1] or 'whatever radically disturbs and upsets the normal order of a person's life'.[2] One person's challenge can be another's crisis or someone else's catastrophe. The same event can be accepted and dealt with by one individual but seem overwhelming and impossible to deal with for another. A crisis is a point at which a person's usual coping skills become inadequate, and it often involves a scenario that is unexpected and has not been met before.

Crisis intervention theory draws quite heavily on the idea of a crisis causing 'disequilibrium' to the client. The client and possibly the client's immediate social system are seen as having to move through intervention towards 'reintegration'.[3] All crisis intervention theorists seem to agree that crisis comes about more readily if a person has not managed past difficulties and so is vulnerable to life stresses or 'hazardous events'. The recommended intervention involves a contract with the client and takes several sessions with a review at the end – what today's mental health services would consider to be a short-term piece of work rather than a swift response to a mental health emergency – but crises can take a period of time to achieve resolution.

Crisis intervention also works on the premise that 'people in crisis are more open to being helped than those who are not'. A person has acknowledged the inadequacy of old coping strategies and so is more likely to be accepting of a fresh formulation of the origin of difficulties and willing to try out new approaches to problem-solving and self-management. It has been pointed out that the Chinese symbol for our word 'crisis' is made up of the two symbols for danger and opportunity.[4] There is danger as the experience of being in crisis can be tortuous, feel unsafe or lead directly to harm to the person. The concept of opportunity may seem insensitive to those in crisis but it is an expression of hope that successful resolution can bring about longer-term benefits.

For the purposes of this book, a mental health crisis occurs when the resources of the client and their social system are insufficient to deal with the events, symptoms or level of distress being experienced and response is needed urgently. It is a set of circumstances which requires a rapid response from somebody external to the usual social system – usually, though not necessarily, mental health services. In receiving any intervention, clients have a right to be supported in their crises in a way which empowers them and their carers to discover new ways to cope. This can in itself work to prevent crises in future.

Following from the above it may seem that we are playing a bit 'fast and loose' with the way we talk about crisis in this book. Crisis intervention purists might feel that our definitions of what are essentially mental health emergencies do not always constitute crisis. However, we would argue that whenever a client (or carers or neighbours or the police etc.) contact a mental health team in need of an urgent response then the situation that client is in has gone beyond what the usual coping strategies of the client and their social system can manage, and *this* constitutes an 'upset in a steady state'.

There are a number of overlaps with the way crisis is classically defined in taking this approach:

- The concept of *disequilibrium* is helpful. The very fact that an urgent response is needed is evidence that disequilibrium has occurred in a client's system or life. If the client and their social system could adjust without outside interference then they would.
- The concept of *danger and opportunity* is relevant to mental health. There is a concern about negative outcomes for the client either from self-harm, loss of liberty or loss of other positives in their life. Conversely, if a person can be assisted to successfully manage a crisis then they are far better placed and more confident to manage future life stresses or severe symptoms (and the two often go together).
- We agree that people are more likely to have difficulties if there are *past unresolved problems*. We use a vulnerability–stress model in approaching mental health crises and past issues that caused distress. This includes not having had the right help to cope with previous times when equilibrium was broken which are self-evidently going to be predisposing factors in

mental health crises. However, we would add other factors that could also make someone vulnerable, discussed later in the chapter.

We do have some differences with the classic theories of crisis work. When mental health services are asked to help a client or a potential client as an emergency then there are some elements that do not apparently fit the theory:

- *The crisis may not be the client's.* The carer or a family member may have a particular life experience, which has either been coming on for a long time or comes out of the blue. This can be what impacts on the client's care and mental health services may be asked to provide alternative support for the client while the carer may choose to deal with their personal crisis with support from elsewhere.
- *The crisis may be about a change in the client's behaviour which is markedly different to their usual behaviour (e.g. an episode of mania).* However, the client may not see that there is a problem and may not welcome assistance. The distress is more likely to be that of the family who are concerned about money being spent, or the client speeding when driving, or about the effect of the mania on relationships.
- *The tenet of crisis resolution, that people are more open to accepting help, is often true, but not necessarily.* Some mental health crises have to be resolved by compulsory intervention under mental health legislation. Having said that, where it is the family who are stressed by the crisis situation and it is not a situation that requires admission for the client, it may be an ideal time to engage with the family and offer suggestions that may help in managing or preventing future episodes if this has not been previously possible.
- *The crisis may not be a new experience.* The theory of crisis envisages a person facing something in life that is new as well as beyond them. Sadly there are many people with mental health problems who have faced similar traumas before. Life changes or stresses that are outside of anyone's control can contribute to the recurrence of symptoms that can be punishing to the client. It may be that with the right sort of help in a crisis the client is better armed to cope the next time, but sometimes people will go through a number of traumatic episodes. It has been said that most people go through crisis once in their life.[5] There are any number of mental health clients whose answer to that would be 'if only'.
- *There are clients who present with mental health emergencies who never seem to reach any equilibrium in their life.* They lurch from problem to problem. They are more likely to be people who have difficulties in coping with their emotions and who may get a diagnosis of personality disorder. In such cases the crisis exists because often the safety of the client is a cause for concern to the extent where it is beyond the control of the client and the client's informal support system. The crisis may be

more about the client being overwhelmed and not coping rather than a radical change in these instances.

So having described our working definition and whether it resembles the classic concept of crisis or not, we can consider what a mental health crisis might actually look like.

What does a mental health crisis look like?

We are going to look at this from two perspectives. The first scenario is when there is no change in the client's symptom level but some change in the social environment puts the client's care in jeopardy and causes the crisis. The second scenario is when, whatever the social triggers, it is the onset, recurrence or worsening of symptoms of mental disorder that the client presents with in crisis.

Although the terms are sometimes used, it is a misnomer to call these 'social and personal' crises. All mental health crises are inevitably social crises because they arise when the problem is too much for the client and their social network to deal with.[6] A client may suffer a horrendous recurrence of symptoms but they will not necessarily be in crisis. It may be that the client can manage with support from family, friends, paid and informal carers, maybe a bit of advice from professionals. Similarly, there may be a breakdown of care arrangements, such as the illness of a carer or the closure of a residential placement. Alternative arrangements may be found that meet the client's needs without too much difficulty and no crisis ensues.

So as all crises are social crises, for the sake of argument we will refer to the two criteria as *situational presentations* and *individual presentations*.

Situational presentations

These can be close to the classic concept of crisis in that they may involve totally new situations that seem beyond the ability of a client or a system to deal with. They may not just involve one client. For example, the closure of a valuable facility or the illness or death of a carer or a project worker in a group home can affect a large number of people, each of whom will respond in their own way. The situation may overlap with individual presentations as a client develops worsening symptoms or else just feels really upset; they need help to build psychological resources to deal with the problem. Or it may be the case that clients are managing well but they are owed a duty of care and new resources need to be found to provide this. Both practical and emotional support is likely to be called for. These crises tend to make up a smaller number of issues that come to the attention of crisis teams.

Individual presentations

These constitute the overwhelming majority of crisis situations seen by mental health teams. They occur when symptoms of mental disorder are evident, usually in response to external stresses or triggers.

People respond to seemingly unbearable stress in different ways. The triggers can come from any number of sources or indeed be a combination of lots of factors. Stressors include the home and family situation, work, occupation or finances, social problems (e.g. falling out with friends), a person's own difficulty finding coping strategies, the pressures of living with racism, homo-phobia, domestic violence or physical illness. Some people have internally-generated stresses reflecting beliefs they have about themselves (e.g. through having unrealistically high expectations of themselves, believing they need to be perfect or always liked – when they do not achieve these states they feel devastated). The list of potential triggers is endless and goes to show how much stress people successfully cope with, without really acknowledging it. However, it is also the case that these triggers can sometimes be changed or worked with to become the resources that will get the person out of the crisis and be used by them to prevent future crises (e.g. perfectionism can be converted into a determination to understand and overcome difficulties).

When people become vulnerable to stress, they may develop or re-experience symptoms of what we call 'mental disorder' and can experience a range of symptoms. We do not use psychiatric diagnoses, as currently formulated, much in this book as clients rarely present with schizophrenia or even anxiety but with symptoms associated with them. Diagnosis is not particularly useful for helping somebody in a crisis as it is of very limited use in management; a person may experience symptoms in a crisis they have never had before and time spent determining diagnosis can be wasted and paralyse or at least limit professionals in thinking about a range of treatment options. It can also have very negative effects on a client's perception of themselves – because the terms used have become stigmatised and misunderstood – and this can lead to arguments, disengagement and disagreements about treat-ment. Unfortunately, our current diagnostic system does not describe causes or predict outcomes to any useful extent and so use of psychiatric diagnoses in crisis management needs to be very carefully handled. If a diagnosis is requested at this stage, careful preparation and discussion of what exactly the diagnosis means – and does not mean – is appropriate. We have chosen in this book to describe individual crises in terms of groups of symptoms or behaviours that present in crisis.

However, it will also be important to draw together the factors involved in leading the person to where they are now. Some type of formulation, making sense of the situation, will need to be drawn up (see Chapter 3). It may then be useful to think about the interactions between the vulnerabilities and strengths, and the stressors and factors that are keeping the problem going.

Patterns can emerge from examining these interactions and in working out a management strategy it may be useful to learn from previous experiences where people have presented with a particular pattern – and if available any evidence of what might work.

The relationship of vulnerability–stress to crisis

Taking an approach which teases out vulnerabilities and acute stresses can be helpful in understanding crises and prioritising the focus of intervention. It may be that the acute issue arises from a loss or threat to the person and specific supports or interventions are needed to cope with it. But the context from which this crisis has developed may shape how successful the intervention is. For example, the threat may be of a partner becoming ill. In this case the context/vulnerability is of dependence on that individual, combined with no previous history of independence.

Some vulnerabilities can be understood but are unchangeable (e.g. a family history of mental health problems). Others are resistant to change (e.g. the individual's personality), whereas others (e.g. social isolation), may have the potential for greater change. However, even those areas that are unchangeable in themselves may have possible implications which can be understood and coped with. For example, someone may have a history of mental health problems in one of their parents and this may have made that person vulnerable through the effects of the family environment or some genetic susceptibility. But more important can be the concern that the problems, which the family member has had, will be inevitably repeated and it is this that causes most distress, usually unnecessarily. Personality characteristics can be vulnerability factors and some may seem resistant to change. However, individual coping strategies can evolve and studies following people with difficulties diagnosed as, say, borderline personality disorder, have shown quite radical change over periods of a decade or more.

Classification can confuse. Does the person have post-traumatic stress disorder (PTSD) or severe depression, borderline personality disorder or psychosis? Unfortunately, these categories seem mutually exclusive when in practice, continua or dual diagnoses exist. Many people with PTSD have the symptoms which are used to diagnose severe depression and many with severe depression have suffered a major traumatic event in their life with degrees of severity of event and of depression occurring. The experiences of flashbacks, voices and in borderline personality disorder (BPD) can seem 'psychotic' and may be so, if the person develops the belief that they are externally generated to themselves. Some patients then also have symptoms of schizophrenia – thought-broadcasting and delusions – which warrant a diagnosis of schizophrenia, while they also have BPD. Diagnostically, attribution may be the key, if internal, i.e. if the thoughts – voices or beliefs – are due to the self and the person's own mind, this suggests BPD; if they are external (e.g. voices are from other people), this suggests psychosis. But of course many patients have difficulty in determining whether very vivid perceptions are internal or external and in practice a continuum exists. Therapeutically, as described later, work with 'psychotic beliefs' and BPD is necessary in sequence and *then* simultaneously.

Understanding the interaction between personality and stressors (including ongoing stressful circumstances) is probably the most useful focus because of the primitive nature of classification. Specific symptoms present as a result and we will use these as an initial guide to presenting alternative routes into working with individuals who may have problems common to wider groups. Classification systems are undergoing review currently, with the World Health Organisation (WHO) and the American Psychiatric Association (APA) focusing on trying to improve validity in the revisions of the *International Classification of Diseases* (ICD11) and the *Diagnostic and Statistical Manual* (*DSM V*). Figure 1.1 illustrates, very simply, some relationships that we have seen in clinical practice between personality, stress and presentations of mental health problems, and some terms that may be helpful (e.g. depression presents in a range of ways with anger, guilt or dependency prominent; psychosis may have apparent roots in trauma, seem drug-related, be due to a marked sensitivity to stress or sometimes converted from anxiety into a 'delusional knowing', where meaning, albeit delusional, alleviates increasing feelings of stress).[7] Many personality categorisations have been proposed over time; the simplest and arguably best validated seems to be

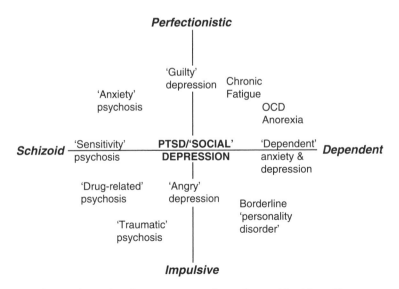

Figure 1.1 Some relationships between personality and mental health problems

that based on extraversion, neuroticism and 'novelty-seeking';[8] in the figure, these essentially relate to schizoid, dependent and perfectionistic-impulsive dimensions.

Professional fear and personal feelings

Before moving on to look at responses to mental health crises, how a mental health professional may *feel* about crisis situations needs consideration. In general, people work in the health and social care services because they have an interest in and/or a concern for others. You are certainly unlikely to hear social workers, nurses, voluntary sector staff and even doctors saying they do the job for the money. But it also needs to be acknowledged that working with people who are in crisis, who have experienced dreadful trauma or who feel desperate, can cause a degree of emotional 'wear and tear' on the practitioner.

A practitioner can easily be drawn into the role of rescuer to resolve their own desire to make everything better. There is also the more serious risk of minimising the client's distress or passing the situation on to others to avoid taking responsibility or time. It is a professional imperative for a practitioner to have an awareness of how they are affected by the crises of others. There is also the need for peer support and management commitment to make this happen. Otherwise, staff become nervous about managing crises and burn out and clients can suffer as a result.

The main fear concerning crises is that of negative outcomes, most commonly the fear that a client may attempt or even complete suicide or harm others if the wrong decision is made or the wrong advice given. The fear is about concern for the client – most staff do care about other people and have a genuine concern to avert any tragedy. But there is also the issue of *blame*. Many staff believe rightly or wrongly that they will be held to account if a client commits suicide. This can be both personal and institutional.

Staff managing crises are usually professionally qualified and accountable for their actions. Clients and their families have the right to expect a good standard of care from services. However, even when staff have done their best and acted professionally, tragedies such as a suicide can occur. On a personal level, some practitioners may blame themselves and apportion themselves a greater responsibility than is rational in what is fundamentally another person's decision to end their life, albeit affected by their mental health problems. On an institutional level, the omnipresence of official inquiries into deaths, serious incidents and 'near-misses' can lead staff to feel they will be blamed for every event that goes, or almost goes, wrong.

The fear of blame leads to defensive practice and can make staff feel quite apprehensive of positive risk-taking. This is frustrating for clients and can hold them back. How is a client with a history of self-harm supposed to believe they can cope if their mental health worker is 'biting their fingernails' about it?

There are personal and institutional responsibilities that are vital to mini-mise a real or perceived 'blame culture' from influencing practice. On a personal level, every practitioner could make an assessment of their own attitude to risk-taking. It does not matter whether a practitioner is by nature a low or a high risk-taker. What matters is that they know that they are a high or a low risk-taker and so can compensate for this in decision-making. Some-body who feels very comfortable taking high risks can then make themselves take note of possible negative outcomes and plan how to manage these. A low risk-taker can consciously examine their own anxiety and look more analytically at the pros and cons of taking risks.

A practitioner's risk-taking attitudes are not fixed over time. Attitudes to risk alter with experience. The suicide of a client can cause a practitioner or a team to be more risk-averse for a period of time through an increase in the fear of another tragedy. There is no shame in this and it is a very understand-able reaction but it is one that should be acknowledged so that other clients' care is not adversely affected.

A positive institutional response to practitioners' concerns about being blamed is needed. Staff need to feel able to discuss concerns with fellow professionals and line managers if and when they need to. For practitioners to be aware of their own feelings, they need adequate, good-quality super-vision from a line manager and time for peer support. A culture where staff feel supported is *crucial*. Decisions about risk should be jointly taken with clients, carers and other members of the care team.

The whole internal inquiry process also needs to be sympathetic and supportive, not accusatory, and staff need to know this will be the case. Then staff can start to look at supporting clients through crises from a position of balance without having to take account of unnecessary increases in their own anxiety as part of the equation. Learning from untoward events is also much more likely to occur.

Relations with clients in crisis can of course be complicated by the staff member's own personal issues and there is a range of excellent books dealing with just these.[9] Very simply, relationships and events in the past and present affect how you react to other people. Understanding and allowing for this enables balanced therapeutic relationships to develop – not doing so can lead to misunderstandings and misjudgements. In everyone's life, relationships with key people (e.g. parents, siblings, partners, even offspring) affect how they relate to people who in some way remind them of these key relationships. The more important the relationship the greater the generalisation from it. Where the relationship has been complicated by difficulties, new relationships can be similarly affected. Therefore it is worth the practitioner considering whether there are similarities between the client and some key individual in the person's life. If so, making allowance for these is vital, ensuring that judgements or reactions are to that person and not transferred from others. Where uncertainty arises or the practitioner or others recognise that reactions to a client seem to be out of proportion or not quite appropriate to the circumstances, reviewing why this might be so with colleagues or a supervisor is worth considering.

Crisis situations can lead to significant distress in staff. Hearing distressing descriptions of the trauma that people have faced, witnessing scenes where they may have to be admitted to hospital or treated against their will, having to face verbal and, on rare occasions, even physical hostility and abuse can leave significant marks. There is a clear obligation on mental health services to make available support and offer appropriate debriefing after such events. The evidence from debriefing studies seems to be that this can have mixed – even negative – results but it can only be humane to ensure that where colleagues have experienced a traumatic incident, they are given time and support to work it through and recover from it.

Chapter 2

Engaging and assessing the client

Engagement and assessment are ongoing processes which start when you first get given information about the client and do not finish until you part from them. Even then you may go on gathering or receiving information which will be relevant to the client's subsequent management. Engagement can also fluctuate and requires focused consideration in relation to your individual relationship with the client and that of the service longer-term. Preparation for meeting the person is very important. We continue with discussion of mapping of available community resources and involvement of carers, safety considerations, engagement issues, full assessment and specific situations (e.g. homeless clients).

Context for assessment

Referrals for assessments in crisis come from a variety of sources. Many are internal NHS referrals from family doctors to mental health teams, or they could be self-referrals or a response to concerns expressed by carers, members of the public or the police. Before any assessment can take place the mental health worker needs to know what the purpose of the assessment is and the context in which it is occurring. Much of the former will be conveyed by the referrer, for example, concern about:

- distress;
- risk;

The referrer most likely does not have:

- expertise;
- time to make assessment;
- resources (e.g access to home treatment teams or inpatient units).

The client and carer may have different perceptions about the reasons for assessment but understanding the referrer's expectations is still important to enable an appropriate response to them.

Assessment takes place within different legislative and social frameworks. In England and Wales, the NHS and Community Care Act 1990 gave social services responsibility for assessing need and coordinating care of adults needing assistance, including adults with mental health problems, on request by them or their carer. The assessment of these clients along with the implementation, monitoring and review of any care provided as a result of the assessment is known as *care management*. This legislation and assessments under it should dovetail in mental health with the Care Programme Approach in England. This was a Department of Health (DoH) response to an inquiry into the murder of a mental health social worker, intended to ensure that people with severe mental illness receive the care and support they need. As with care management, one mental health practitioner (described as the client's 'care coordinator') has the lead responsibility for a client's assessment(s), drawing up a care plan with them and coordinating and monitoring delivery of their care and support in the community with regular review.[1,2] There are also times when assessments take place under mental health legislation when compulsory admission is being contemplated as an option.

As well as the various functions of the assessment and different referral routes, there are also different professions working within mental health teams who undertake assessments – mental health nurses, social workers, occupational therapists, psychiatrists and psychologists. Each profession is likely to have its own approach to assessment dependent on the profession's theories, value base and historic functions. Some of the assessment functions above will be more familiar to some professionals than others. Individuals from different professional backgrounds are therefore likely to approach assessment from radically different angles. For example, although a psychiatrist and a social worker assessing a client in crisis would both take essential personal and family information and look at triggers for the crisis, the psychiatrist may spend more time on medical information and a mental state examination while a social worker may concentrate more on the social circumstances of the client and where the stresses and supports lie within their social framework.

A good assessment in a crisis uses key elements of practice from the range of disciplines represented in mental health services. In our approach to assessment below we examine the individual, familial and wider social factors that it is necessary to understand in order to comprehend what is happening to the client in crisis. There are then some supplementary suggestions for consideration if there is time available or to be discussed on follow-up visits when an individual assessment can be checked out and elaborated upon.

The checking out is in itself very important. 'Lip service' gets paid to the fact that good *assessment is a process not an event*, but this is not always true in practice. A critical observation of initial assessments has noticed that they can assume 'the status of "truth" and become the key determinant to future action and outcomes'.[3] The model and approach we use in assessment may vary according to organisational view and clinical profession. The fact remains that we are only presenting a version of the situation at that time. It is for this reason that the sharing and checking of the assessment with the client becomes so important, as is continuing to be open to new information and changes in circumstances and presentation.

Sources of information

The primary source will initially be the referrer and then the client themselves, but secondary sources can provide vital information before the assessment begins (see Box 2.1), and later. It does not breach confidentiality to receive information from other sources (see Chapter 3) – there need not even be an admission that the person is undergoing assessment. Information may be offered spontaneously by family or friends or others but may need to be sought. This will be the case in the crisis situation where the client is incommunicative or what they say is difficult to understand.

Basic information needs to be gathered before the assessment is agreed with the referrer and begins (see Box 2.2). Many services will already have a

---

Box 2.1 Sources of information

These include:

- reports from the individual themselves;
- families or other carers;
- friends;
- neighbours;
- staff who've known them previously;
- previous psychiatric records, manual and computerised;
- records from other sources (where available and accessible and, generally, with the client's permission);
- family doctors;
- other medical notes;
- social workers (e.g. from children and family or physical disability teams);
- criminal records or statements from the police;
- local newspapers where circumstances of specific reported events are relevant;
- professional observations of body language and environmental changes.

Box 2.2 Information for crisis referral needed from referrer

- Referrer's details: name, address, contact telephone.
- Client's details: name, address, age/date of birth.
- Urgency: degree (immediate, hours, days) and reasons for referral.
- Where do they want them seen.
- Presenting problem: duration and current treatment.
- Risks: current and past.
- Past history: when, what happened, what treatment.
- Any specific expectations by referrer of the assessment.
- Anything else relevant (e.g. need for interpreter, gender issues).

---

proforma available for this purpose. In practice, a balance will need to be struck between seeking all the information that can be obtained and that which is necessary to ensure risks are assessed and managed effectively so that duplication of previous assessments is kept to an appropriate level. Unnecessary delay in seeing the client can prolong their distress and increase risks. However, you will need to ensure that your service is the correct one to act upon the referral and that the situation does constitute a crisis and requires immediate action. As discussed in Chapter 9, a range of mental health teams now exist, many taking direct referrals, and there is considerable room for overlap. This can improve the service offered to the client but also increase the potential for gaps to emerge. There may also be circumstances where physical symptoms (see Chapter 8) suggest the need for medical interventions initially. In these circumstances, the referrer can be asked to negotiate an assessment with another team but, certainly if there are likely to be differences of opinion, you may need to obtain agreement on who needs to make an assessment. If in doubt or where negotiations are becoming protracted, making an initial direct assessment, possibly jointly with the referrer or worker from another relevant service, is generally safest. The situation can be assessed and stabilised, and any long-term involvement needed can be negotiated under less pressure.

Where to assess?

Not everybody is going to have the luxury of choice in this matter. There are constraints of time for most practitioners or of location for others (e.g. a practitioner may be restricted to seeing clients in certain venues such as a hospital, clinic or accident and emergency department because of the need to provide cover to that particular site. If you have a choice and the client is agreeable, the most comprehensive and effective assessment will almost always be in the client's home environment. We make an assessment on the basis of what the client tells us, what others tell us and what we observe about the client and their surroundings.

If the client is on home territory they are likely to be more relaxed and able to speak. It is more likely that the assessing practitioner will meet the family or the client's friends and so can make an assessment of the level of informal social support the client has. It is invaluable to know if someone's family is supportive, anxious or overtly hostile. Environment is also a clue to the level of mental health difficulty. A client may *say* they are coping but a home which is looking far less tidy than usual, with no evidence of the client having eaten for example, could indicate they are struggling and provide clues as to a line of discussion regarding possible self-neglect.

Some clients will not want a home visit if they do not want the conversation overheard or if they feel it is an invasion of their privacy. Clients may also feel embarrassed if their home has become neglected in their eyes. These views should be respected where possible. There may also be risk issues in visiting a client at home (see Chapter 4) and these should obviously be taken into account when deciding on the appropriate venue.

Carers and advocates in assessments

Some practitioners have strong feelings about seeing clients on their own during an assessment, often because of well-intentioned fears that carers will speak on the client's behalf or inhibit what the client feels able to say. However, the decision as to whether the carer is part of the assessment process should be the client's as far as possible. A client can certainly be asked, while on their own, about what they want (e.g. somebody who suffers domestic violence will not want that aggressor in their mental health assessment or a client using illegal drugs may not want the family to know this). However, a client is in a powerless situation when being assessed and should be offered the option of having a carer, friend or advocate sit in. If the carer or friend talks for the client, it is easy enough to ask them not to do so, although it may be necessary to repeat and reinforce this. The only reasons for not allowing a carer to be present could be if they pose a risk to the practitioner (e.g. by being intimidating) or are oppressive to the client.

For assessments under mental health legislation in the UK currently, the Code of Practice states that if the 'patient wants or needs another client (e.g. a friend, relative or an advocate) to be present during the assessment and any subsequent action that may be taken then ordinarily the ASW [coordinating practitioner] should assist in securing that client's attendance unless the urgency of the case or some other reason makes it inappropriate to do so'.[4] This formalises what we consider to be good practice in all crisis assessments.

If a practitioner is seeing the client alone, it is important to ensure that relatives or others accompanying them are also interviewed, possibly by a colleague, with the client's permission. Alternatively they could be asked to wait to be seen or at worst a mobile or other phone contact and name could be taken. This may also apply to emergency services that may have very relevant information about the circumstances of being called out. Friends or relatives can provide invaluable information and also further support to the client.

Community care and community mapping

Any assessment of an individual takes place within a social context. It is part of the preparation for assessment that background information about the client's community becomes important. This is not work to be done when the referral comes in but should be a pool of knowledge built up over time to be shared by mental health teams and the localities they serve. Practitioners can draw on this information when making assessments.

In discussing community care there is often very little said about what constitutes the community and not enough emphasis placed on defining the community within which the client is being offered care. This can be particularly the case in health-led Community Mental Health Teams which may tend to work more from a culture of therapeutic alliances with individuals rather than with a client's social environment.

The point of assessment is to find out what you need to know in order to offer assistance to the client being assessed, either via service provision or else via advice and referral on. It is also about discovering what strengths the client has that can be utilised to overcome the presenting problem. It is common practice therefore in any mental health assessment to ask about the client's family in order to identify whether there are stresses within the family and to look at who in the family can help in a carer role or as a distraction from the client's distress.

The idea behind community mapping is that there is no need to stop at discussing just the individual and the family. We all live in society and the more we are engaged in the multiple communities that surround us, the more scope we all have to access support, interests, distractions and a sense of belonging that mitigates against the feelings of isolation that mental health problems can leave people with.

There are broadly speaking two types of community: *geographical communities* and *communities of interest*. Communities of interest are defined by the individual and it can be a useful exercise to map your own. This would involve looking at the groups of people you mix with or have contact with, even at a superficial level, on a regular basis. For a client seeking help in a potential crisis, a few questions about how they spends their time might reveal the following:

Ayesha

- Age 30.
- People in her block of flats – minimal contact.
- Day centre, mum and kids groups or depression group.
- Part-time job in local shop – work colleagues.
- Family – child, age 3.
- Playgroup mums and kids.
- Auntie and uncle, one sister.
- Local church, regular attender if well.
- Social and political background – some stigma as a lone parent.

The prospect for Ayesha accessing community support is good. She has support via a day centre and can call on social contacts from work, worship and leisure for support or distractions without being over-reliant on any one support. There may be psychological barriers to her accessing her communities, but these are much easier to work on when the communities are in place to be utilised.

A less well networked client may have a smaller range of communities of interest:

Bob

- Age 55.
- People in local shops – say hello at most.
- People in street – say hello at most.
- Two old friends, occasional contact.
- Local pub regulars – heavy drinkers.
- Family – two sons, live far away, divorced.
- Social and political background – long-term sick on benefits, little disposable income, less social and occupational opportunities.

Bob has less to call on. His contacts may well encourage him to drink heavily and this risks exacerbating his mental health difficulties. So in looking at crisis prevention with Bob, the development of community involvement would help. It is therefore vital to know what communities of interest there are and how they can be accessed.

The practitioners at the greatest disadvantage here are those new to the locality and doctors in training and other temporary staff (e.g. from agencies) as they move so frequently it is practically impossible to build up an adequate picture of local resources. There is a responsibility on the local mental health service to compile information for the benefit of those practitioners who are new and short-term and a responsibility on the part of these staff to ask for this.

In mental health teams, information is always available about communities of mental health interest, such as day centres or MIND clubs. There is usually information about drug and alcohol services. More variable are the projects, places and activities going on in the geographical community. Mental health practitioners rarely get the opportunity to properly profile the geographical community they serve; much of the information in teams is piecemeal and anecdotal. However, if information is put together, a fairly useful geographical community profile can be constructed. Within a particular patch there can be many community opportunities available (see Box 2.3).

Practitioners can use knowledge learnt from clients regarding how the community can support or cause stress to an individual or family. Some estates have thriving facilities, others may be known for drug problems or poor lighting. Being aware of the public transport systems in the area is crucial for service provision at both planning and access levels. If you know your area, you know what your client may have to contend with in the way of extra stresses and difficulties but also what activity is going on around the client that they can be supported to tap into.

Box 2.3 Community resources

- Social clubs.
- Volunteering opportunities.
- Advice centres.
- Detached youth workers.
- Youth centres.
- Community cafés.
- Volunteering agencies.
- Parent and toddler groups.
- Play schemes.
- Libraries.
- Toy libraries.
- Leisure and sports centres.
- Adult education.
- Parks.
- Places of worship (all faiths).
- Community centres.

Local newspapers may also list local associations offering specialist help. The internet is an instant source of information about national or less well-known organisations to meet a need or an interest.

This gives a context for your assessments. Clients presenting for help do not just carry difficulties and solutions inside themselves. Other difficulties and solutions can lie inside their social milieu.

Pre-assessment safety issues

The final pause for thought prior to assessment is about the health and safety issues for the practitioner and the client. The concerns for staff are verbal abuse, environmental hazards, feeling alone in an unknown area and also physical violence (see Chapter 4). The concerns for the client are similar, although they may expect staff not to be verbally abusive or violent. However, previous experiences of being forcibly removed to hospital can give rise to fears of being subjected to physical force. If people feel threatened, there is a much lower chance of a productive conversation between them.

There may be risks associated with assessing the client in a particular environment. The client may have no history of violence but they may share accommodation with people who do. There are environmental risks in some areas such as needle stick injuries if the client or their housemates use drugs intravenously. It may be that the client lives in an area known for pub 'closing time' violence and the assessment is a night-time emergency callout.

As part of the assessment preparation, questions can be asked of the referrer about risk issues. A family doctor can be asked if there is a history of violence from the client and their family and the surgery is likely to have an idea of locality risk issues. Out of hours the police are available for advice where sufficient suspicion arises. For previously-known clients there should be pertinent information on any computer warning screens or databases or in health or social service notes. However the absence of such information about risk does not mean risk does not exist.

If a client or somebody living with the client is known or even suspected to pose a potential risk to others then a plan of how to assess safely needs careful thought. This is also the case when the common situation arises that nothing is known about the person who is to be seen. At the very least, with a risk of just verbal assault, consideration should always be given to two practitioners attending.

Could the assessment take place in a safer environment, for example a hospital or mental health centre? However this in itself does not provide automatic protection and other plans can be made to reduce the risk. There are ways to acknowledge anger, remaining respectful and using empathy. Skilled practitioners will also be alert to body language during assessment, their own and the client's, and the use that can be made of the seating arrangements for a non-confrontational atmosphere. There needs to be the facility to get help quickly via a panic button and, at the most extreme, police back-up may be needed. Every interview environment therefore needs seats (although sometimes even these are not available), privacy – as far as this is compatible with safety – an alarm and usually a phone (possibly a mobile, charged up and with a strong signal).

Other questions to consider might be whether the choice of personnel visiting alters the level of risk (e.g. is the risk posed to a particular gender of worker?). Or it may be that a particular member of staff is feeling threatened. If the assessment is essential and the client will not attend an office base then the police should be asked to assist. The nature of the risk should be made clear to the police as well as exactly what role they are being asked to play. They may be asked to wait outside or may need to be present during the assessment. Use of the police inevitably affects the tone of the assessment and can work powerfully against engagement. Practitioners can explain and apologise for a police presence, for example by saying that 'Our records indicate that you have assaulted a member of staff when unwell and drinking in the past so now we have to err on the side of caution and be accompanied by the police for our safety. We are sorry this looks so heavy handed.' Such explanations given in a non-judgemental tone can make clear the police presence is not intended to threaten the client, however it is still likely to feel that way to the person being assessed. They may dispute the evidence from the records and while this will be worth discussing, caution will usually dictate that the level of support be maintained.

The key point about managing the risks in assessment is that practitioners are not left alone. Assessment should be a team effort, both in deciding how to manage the difficulties while retaining maximum respect for the client and in carrying out that decision: 'Everyone involved in assessment should be alert to the need to provide support for colleagues, especially where there is a risk of the patient causing physical harm'.[5]

What if the client refuses assessment?

This may be their right and after gathering what information is available and assessing the risks involved, it may be decided that assessment cannot proceed. Assessing the client's capacity to make this decision is probably wise (see Chapter 3). Any decision not to proceed needs to be discussed with the referrer if possible and the position of any carer or person being cared for by them also needs to be considered. They may need to be given help in their own right or at least a contact telephone number to use if circumstances change. It can be worth outlining the type of changes that would warrant making contact again (e.g. the client describes suicidal thoughts to the carer, or their behaviour becomes increasingly strange, or the situation does not resolve itself within a given time).

Considerations may need to be given to using a warrant under mental health legislation to obtain access if a client is not agreeable to the assessment and there is evidence that grounds for compulsory assessment exist.[6] The police in most countries have powers to take a person from a public place to a designated 'place of safety' which can be a police station or health premises where they can ask for an assessment to be conducted. Such compulsory assessments will be more difficult because the person, understandably, may express objections to this happening and is often more difficult to engage with. In such circumstances it can be difficult to distinguish these objections from the expression of paranoid ideas.

Engaging the client

How does the client feel about assessment?

Before approaching any assessment a practitioner needs to think about what the assessment means to the client. Has the client been desperate for help or is the client seeing you reluctantly (as just discussed) at somebody else's request? Initial thoughts about how to engage with the client can make for a more relaxed discussion. It may involve apologising to the client if they have waited for a long time to be seen or thanking the reluctant client for agreeing to see you.

Being assessed by a mental health practitioner can be a nerve-wracking experience, particularly to somebody who is new to services or who has past experience of compulsory admission. For a new client, all they may have are ideas about psychiatry and related services derived from the media.

Although we may like to see ourselves as caring, sensitive individuals, clients may not have that expectation and anxiety can be high. A further fear for a client can be that they may not receive a service they want as a result of the assessment (or they may get a service they don't want, possibly involving the use of the mental health legislation). We need to be aware that our presence could be heightening distress.

With all patients, engagement is the essential first stage of contact although usually this is accompanied or rapidly followed by assessment. Maintaining engagement is critically important and there are a range of issues which impinge upon this. The setting you meet in is important, as discussed earlier. Risk issues need consideration (see above and Chapter 4) and availability of time is also relevant such that a judgement needs to be made about how critical the venue for the meeting is. Sometimes where the first meeting is difficult in a mental health centre or office elsewhere, offering a second at the person's home can be positive.

Personal appearance is important and it is worth considering how you present to others. Are you relaxed, casual, sloppy or pristine? You can't change your appearance to suit every patient but you can be aware of the possible impact on them. Language can also have variable effects: too complex a vocabulary can lead to lack of understanding; too simple can lead to the client feeling patronised. Noting non-verbal responses and using brief summaries and regular feedback can elucidate this. If you use technical terms, it's essential they are understood – talking at the level the person understands is essential.

Interaction involves the development of trust and collaboration. Clients presenting in crisis are usually at a point in their lives when they are inviting engagement and asking for support so this can be an opportunity to commence or improve a relationship with an individual mental health practitioner and mental health services as a whole. It is also an occasion when unsympathetic and ineffective actions can alienate the client – first impressions can be very important. Straightforward, competent approaches can therefore lead to effective engagement on which to build collaborative assessment and intervention in the crisis and prevention strategies for the future.

Crisis presentations may involve reluctance or ambivalence on the part of the client, even antagonism where they don't believe they have a problem or, at least, that mental health services are not appropriate for dealing with any issues they have. Engagement in these circumstances remains of primary importance but can be difficult to achieve. However, developing some degree of collaboration is necessary for assessment and intervention if involuntary measures are to be avoided.

Anxious and depressed clients will frequently engage readily and assessment and intervention can proceed. However, those with behavioural presentations, eating disorders and psychosis may be trickier. With the latter and others with whom forming a relationship is an issue, specific attention to engagement is worth considering. Often we take developing a therapeutic relationship for granted, simply acting intuitively, which may not be sufficient to begin or maintain engagement.

Where engagement is an issue, it essentially overrides any other consideration (with the exception of immediate attention to threats to self or others). If assessment or interventions are interfering with engagement, as opposed to facilitating it, there may need to be:

- a reconsideration of the way assessment is proceeding or how interventions are being used;
- diversion to issues with which the client is more comfortable, for a period;
- a brief period of relaxed conversation about non-clinical subjects;
- a pause to retain and enhance engagement – sometimes it may be possible to break off to drink a cup of tea before recommencing.

The client may walk out of the assessment and consideration needs to be given immediately as to the appropriate action:

- If risks have been assessed as immediately present, it may be necessary to go with them and continue the assessment 'on foot'.
- If they refuse or try to run away, it may be necessary to restrain them but only if appropriate trained support is available (see Chapter 4).

- It may be worth walking with them to continue the assessment even if risks are not currently apparent. This can be the case where there are quite a lot of people involved and the client feels overwhelmed, or where disagreements with the carer occur. Another room, the garden or a park bench may make suitable alternative venues. For others involved in the assessment, keeping within calling distance, even where risks are deemed low, is a sensible precaution.
- The client can often be allowed to leave, conversation can continue with the carer or others involved and very frequently the client will return or the interview is reconvened later.

Engagement can be a major obstacle with people suffering from personality disorders or severe mental illness, especially where paranoia is prominent, but there are ways forward (see the case example below).

Martin had a history of paranoid schizophrenia with abuse of amphetamines and was very distrustful of authority and mental health services. He presented in crisis to a duty worker at the local mental health centre with a list of demands and complaints about the response of services to his needs. By working through these individually and developing a collaborative approach to medication management, in particular, a relationship gradually developed enabling him to leave the initial interview in a more relaxed and accepting frame of mind. He later engaged with longer-term work looking at and working with relevant issues.

Effective engagement emphasises collaboration, warmth and mutual respect. From the perspective of the client who might be distressed by symptoms such as recurrent panic attacks, accusatory auditory hallucinations, experiences of thought insertion or persecutory fears, especially where interactions with services have not been helpful, it may take time to begin to build trust within any form of therapeutic interaction. Engagement varies from client to client and some of the factors which enhance and impair it include cultural similarity and difference, accent, language, vocabulary (match to the individual), tone of voice, trying not to talk down to them, and pace and volume of speech.

Taking account of these factors can assist in determining the necessary tactics used. It may seem pedantic to say that communication needs to be between equals as far as possible but it is a frequent complaint from users of services that they do not feel respected. This is not to neglect the power imbalances that exist – the mental health practitioner may have advantages of class, experience, control of access to services and the ability to impose treatment if certain circumstances exist, but nevertheless respect between two individuals should still be sought. Respect for the client's beliefs, however seemingly negative, bizarre or irrational, may be difficult but should be possible. These beliefs have meaning to them and it is rare for the ideas expressed not be understandable when the context in which they developed is known. Staff often have difficulties with understanding clients' behaviour and this may be associated with difficulties in supporting such mutual respect, for example:

- Self-harm is often described as 'manipulative', yet if it is understood as a very effective, albeit short-term, way for the individual to reduce distress that they are finding intolerable, it can be *understood*. For example, an overdose dulls emotional distress quickly and cutting can provide relief of overwhelming feelings of tension and self-blame.
- Antisocial behaviour can have many origins (e.g. a learned response to stress, intolerance of frustration, or for gain). It is also a significant risk factor for mental health problems and harm to self or others. Understanding the client's reasoning underlying their behaviour can help address these issues even if the behaviour itself cannot be sanctioned. A relationship which respects the individual human being with their complexities, strengths and vulnerabilities, can enable assessment, engagement and appropriate intervention. This relationship in itself can be a therapeutic tool in relation to the mental health problems and antisocial behaviour (see Chapter 6).

In situations where engagement is proving particularly difficult, the notion of 'befriending' can be valuable. It simply means acting as a friend would to the client (as far as that is possible in a professional relationship). As an intervention, befriending provides human contact with a focus on discussing neutral but engaging topics, such as holidays, the weather, sport or TV. It has also proved valuable when disengagement appears to be occurring – something said or assumed by the client has upset the relationship – or distressing events have been broached and led to an increase in agitation. Shifting into conversational chat can often retrieve a situation, allowing a return to significant issues later. An openness to discuss a wide range of concepts and philosophies (everything from existentialism to human biology, witchcraft to astrophysics) can improve engagement as can taking an interest in any such material produced by the client. Even though statements may seem to be part of symptomatology, exploring them may be a way of explaining and understanding the odd feelings and thoughts that the client is experiencing. It may seem that such discussion has no place in crisis care because of the restricted time available and the necessity of dealing with so many other issues. However, our experience is the reverse – that directly engaging with what the client wants to discuss can be a key part of assessment and engagement, building cooperation in order to explore risk and develop subsequent management issues rapidly and effectively.

All practitioners need the core skills of empathy and active listening.

Encounters with people presenting in crisis should aim to include elements common to working with anybody: genuineness, openness and unconditional positive regard – respect for the client and their symptoms. Warmth and humour are often helpful. This type of approach allows sessions to be enjoyable for both parties and can make difficult issues easier to discuss and action points more memorable. It also allows the client to stand back from their symptoms and look at alternatives without 'losing face'. Humour needs to be used carefully, especially if someone is overtly distressed, oversensitive or paranoid. If humour could be misconstrued as laughing or smiling *at* the client rather than *with* them, it may be better to avoid using it. Often the prompt leading to laughter or a smile comes from the client themselves and can be reciprocated and even added to or amplified.

The pace of the initial interview needs to be considered carefully. The process can be slow where concentration is poor or symptoms interfere. When the assessment and management plan is slowly-paced, paradoxically the client often makes steady, sometimes even rapid progress; however, attuning the pace of progress to the individual works best. When the client is hesitant, rephrasing questions may assist but it remains very important to allow sufficient time for the client to process the question given and arrive at a reply. Often responses are affected by distraction originating from depressive, psychotic or other symptoms. The client may be experiencing voices or thinking about paranoid, anxious or depressive beliefs. For example, if they fear that the police are outside waiting to arrest them, they may be understandably reluctant to answer your questions; similarly if their main concern is to get 'proper' medical attention for their physical symptoms. This may be because they see your questions as being irrelevant to their situation (see Chapter 8). On the other hand, silence can be anxiety-provoking and long periods of this are better avoided – keeping the flow of conversation going in a relaxed fashion is generally most effective at building a relationship.

Whether you take notes as you speak with the client depends on your style and available time. For most busy practitioners, it is almost inevitable that they will have to take notes as they proceed. Notes may also be a more accurate record of the conversation and of risk issues and are immediately available when the interview is finished, especially if this occurs prematurely. This can be useful where the client is going to hospital or leaving with another health or social care professional. Writing a record afterwards has the advantage of allowing you to concentrate, and appear to concentrate, fully on what the client is telling you and so can enhance engagement. It can also lead to a clearer, more legible and better-organised account. It can be worth checking with the client what their views are about this and taking these into account or at least explaining why you are writing notes. Certainly if the client asks you not to write, as sometimes occurs, it is best at least to pause to discuss the specific issue involved unless there are very good reasons to continue. Where the client is talking about particularly sensitive or distressing issues, discontinuing writing for that period is also courteous and considerate.

Interactions with people with mental health problems (e.g. psychosis and especially behavioural problems) can become confrontational or conversely collusive or patronising. Unfortunately such interactions lead to increased isolation of the client and to symptom maintenance. Patients stop reporting their symptoms to staff members when this happens. On the other hand, a client with mental health problems, especially psychosis, may not be used to being given sufficient time to voice their ideas and concerns, and when given the opportunity to do so is often very interested in the assessor's attitudes and opinions. The way in which the assessor expresses them can be pivotal. Accurate and consistent responses can move the relationship to a position where assessment and work on explanatory models and a management plan can occur. This may mean avoiding platitudes such as 'You'll get better' or collusion with beliefs, particularly psychotic ones whilst answering questions raised by the client effectively. For example:

Client: You don't believe the police are after me do you?
Practitioner: What you have told me so far has made it clearer to me why you think they are after you. I'm just not so sure myself at the moment. So do you want to tell me a bit more or maybe we can come back to this later.

Apparent incomprehensibility of a client's symptoms can lead to an impasse which affects further intervention. If the practitioner is able to demonstrate the expectation that the symptoms will make sense in due course, trust can be developed. In the same way that anxiety, depression and phobias are psychologically understandable in terms of their formulation and content, so it now seems (from the success of cognitive behaviour therapy (CBT) in schizophrenia) are the various symptoms of psychoses. This may be difficult to believe for the practitioner (especially a psychiatrist) who is new to this way of working, but further experience of working with people with psychosis is usually convincing.

Lack of response altogether can occur. This can be through non-cooperation and a decision about whether the assessment should continue needs to be taken. It can be because of paranoia, mutism, stupor, fear or negative symptoms. With each of these, gentle questioning or sometimes diversionary discussion about what is happening, explaining why the assessment is occurring, trying to allay fears or anger, sometimes even discussion of something which you think might engage their attention – sport, TV – allows some form of assessment to occur even if it is only of non-verbal responses which in turn may open up conversation. Initially this can simply be question and nod/shake head or yes/no answers but may develop from there.

If there is a gradual or sudden increase in agitation or distress in relation to any particular line of questioning or investigation it is generally better to suggest moving away and offering to return to this area later. Often talk about less distressing areas or befriending topics can reduce the tension so that the interview progresses and is terminated amicably. Where differences emerge and the client becomes confrontational with the practitioner, 'agreeing to differ' is a non-confrontational way out which allows a return to the subject matter later or a different approach to be taken. For example: 'I can see how important this issue is to you and that we are having problems agreeing about exactly what all this means. Perhaps we could agree to differ and talk about other important matters. It'll give me some time to think about it so we can talk about it later or when we meet again' (or, if more appropriate, 'when you see your care coordinator, therapist, the ward nurses, psychiatrist' etc.).

Engagement with clients from other cultural groups can be particularly problematic and style, process and content may be relevant. Style can differ in terms of language, tone, accent, etc., and explanations given for symptoms may differ. The ideal therefore may be to have a practitioner from the client's own culture – but that may significantly restrict members of some cultures from receiving the appropriate levels of expert intervention because of the limited availability of trained and experienced practitioners. Perhaps the most practical way of handling this difficult issue is to accept that cross-cultural therapy is inevitable but that this needs to be discussed explicitly and opportunities provided for the client to have an advocate or practitioner from their own background to reassess them as soon as is possible. If it is agreed that cross-cultural assessment and intervention will occur, involvement of advocates, friends or carers in support and to interpret cultural implications, and an interpreter, if required, may help. However, the client needs to be able to choose whether this will be helpful or not. Families may have their own interpretations and needs which can lead to complications and adversely affect assessment and the subsequent intervention and crisis planning. Sometimes communication can be impaired by accent or limited language capacity and this can become frustrating and even increase paranoia. The assessor may not want to interrupt the client but has difficulty understanding them and vice versa, and so misunderstandings can arise. Repeated interruptions can restrict the flow of narrative. Negotiating ways of communicating effectively (e.g. speaking more slowly), with regular feedback and summarising can help.

Gender is also an issue to consider and it is important not to presume that 'good practice' can automatically accommodate gender issues. Some men and women can talk and trust people of the same, or occasionally opposite, gender more easily. This issue is especially important where sexual or relationship issues are central to therapy, or where issues relating to current male or female roles in society are relevant. Again, it is best to allow choice where possible, and to reassess if progress is not made. Offering accommodation for a client's choices in the future may be helpful where choice cannot be offered immediately. Sometimes women or men will refuse to see someone of a particular gender and this can cause significant practical difficulties. The reason may be known or suspected (e.g. previous assaults or abuse or the nature of current difficulties), or unknown. There are some alternative steps that can be tried:

- The risks of deferring full assessment until this issue can be resolved may need to be determined. The distress entailed in delay will also influence this decision. If deferment is necessary, it may involve agreeing an alternative time and place for assessment with a male or female practitioner as requested or establishing a protective environment at home or in a crisis house or hospital until the assessment can be completed.
- A telephone consultation with a colleague elsewhere who can assist in determining risk, at least, and sometimes more information and an interim crisis plan may be a solution.
- The client can be offered support during the interview from a male or female friend, carer or support worker.

Finally there are a variety of other groups who may have specific issues which need to be taken into account. People who substance misuse or have personality disorders are examples (see Chapter 6). Paranoia can also be expected to interfere; where this is prominent, it may be advisable to use befriending and other ways of developing the therapeutic relationship before much therapy work, even assessment and formulation, is done. However, paradoxically, this may increase paranoia so an initial discussion of how the paranoia has developed may be most appropriate.

Seeing the client

Much has been written about models of assessment but when you have your client sitting down with you, theories of assessment can feel a bit far-removed. In a crisis, there is not always the luxury of time and a number of sessions to do an elongated piece of work. Questioning models of assessment have been criticised[7] for not 'increasing choice, maintaining independence and maximising people's potential'. An 'exchange' model has been advocated as it sees client and professional working in partnership, sharing solutions, with exchanges of information being the tool for assessment. It is a model which puts the client in the role of expert in their own problems instead of the professional. However, and after some soul-searching, for the client in a mental health crisis, we will have to live with the use of questions. It is naïve and self-deceptive for professionals to pretend that the power imbalance in the assessment process is not present and active. Some clients are seeing the mental health worker under compulsion and probably many more with some reluctance. The worker does have the power to say yes or no to service provision for the client or family in distress. The worker may have the power to recommend detention under mental health legislation. It is not an equal power relationship. Having made this explicit, this very imbalance puts certain obligations on the mental health worker at the start of the assessment.

What to discuss with the client initially

The client has a right to know:

- what is about to happen during the assessment;
- the names and roles of everyone present (in a Mental Health Act assessment there can be quite a gathering of people);
- the boundaries of confidentiality;
- what the range of likely outcomes could be (e.g. a service, no service, compulsory detention, home treatment and some information about service criteria);
- information that you have already and why you are there.

It is also the responsibility of the mental health worker, being aware of their relational power, to try to work against this imbalance to make the assessment as comfortable for the client as possible. This includes making efforts not to be oppressive in language or behaviour, being respectful and acknowledging any gaps in their own knowledge – for example, if you have no knowledge of a client's religious or cultural background, admit this and ask for advice if needed.

The presence of trainee nurses, doctors and social workers at assessments needs a mention. They have much to gain from attending such assessments but their involvement needs to be discussed with the client before they are invited to be present. This is not always easy in practice but is essential – the client should not be put in a position where they have to refuse with the trainee present. The trainee can always be asked to leave the room or site where the assessment is taking place so that this can be established. The client should also be made aware that they can ask the trainee to leave at any time and sometimes, if the assessor thinks that the presence of the trainee is an issue (e.g. very sensitive material is being disclosed and the client gives perhaps non-verbal indications of their discomfort with the trainee being present) they may request them to leave. The client also needs to be assured that they have every right not to have a trainee present and will not be penalised in any way if they decide against. It is also important that the trainee is aware of their role, i.e. observer, in this setting. Risk issues also need assessment. Where risks to the assessing team exist but nevertheless the assessment has to proceed, involvement of trainees is unlikely to be appropriate except for experienced practitioners who are training to upgrade their qualifications and are already skilled.

Inviting the client to tell their story

The areas to be considered are broadly:

- the client's individual problems, presenting physical and mental health problems and past history;
- their family, friends and domestic arena;
- their community and social environment;
- the wider political issues affecting the above.

The client's individual current problems

The client needs to be given some time initially to describe in their own words what they see the situation to be and what the crisis is. Once the client has told you this, it is possible to start to fill in any gaps. How they specifically describe their current problems and situation is important (e.g. 'I've nowhere to live', 'I'm frightened I'm going to die', 'there are people who won't stop following me'). Other necessary information includes how these particular problems developed, when they started, what was involved and how the problems are affecting the client and those around them.

There are also background areas that should be covered in a good assessment. Sometimes, especially in crisis, clients may need explanations as to why we want to discuss these areas which may seem irrelevant. Such explanations include saying that this allows you to understand them and their current circumstances better and how to best find helpful ways of dealing with the current crisis.

History of mental health problems

This is important as it gives clues as to how someone may have managed crises in the past. Does the client have a history of admissions, community or GP treatment for mental health problems? When and where was this? Was it for similar problems (e.g. particular self-harming behaviour, or a pattern of relapse in response to certain known stressors)? Is there a history of actions or thoughts leading to significant risk to themselves or others? It is also vital to obtain information on the client's current medication and any information they can share on the effects of past medication: what they think has helped and what hasn't or has caused problematic side-effects. You may have this information if you have past records in front of you but that isn't always possible and, even when it is, the client's perceptions are often not noted. There are also frequently interventions or coping methods that have helped apart from medication which it is useful to know about.

There is no need to assume that history will always repeat itself, so a client's current presentation should not be invalidated by past events. For example, if a client does not have a history of acting on suicidal thoughts it cannot be assumed that they never will. Similarly if a client has always used acute inpatient care to manage crises in the past there should still be careful thought given to supporting the client in community-based care if that is achievable with the client's wishes taken into account.

Understanding personal and family history

It is not always possible to assess family and personal history in crisis situations but where it can be done it is valuable. If the client is not prepared to talk about it or if they are currently threatening themselves or other people and immediate action is necessary, the previously-mentioned areas may be the only information that can be gathered. However, often information is available through previous records or from other people to allow a fuller picture to be drawn.

Building on the information supplied above, it can be useful to ask about parents and other family members (brothers, sisters and others with whom they have contact or are influential on them, e.g. grandparents). Where are they, what contact do you have, what's the relationship been like? As discussed below, they may be available to provide support or further information. An understanding of relationships with significant others can influence the management plan. For example, abusive or unsupportive relationships or recent bereavement may have negative implications.

A client history – a brief story of their life – might seem too much to ask of a client in crisis but often clients will provide a brief synopsis of this and it can illuminate their current situation for you and them. It becomes clearer why they are, for example, panicking about physical symptoms when you learn that they have had a number of bereavements or been very affected by someone else's illness in the past. Where were they born and bought up? Did they have any problems early on in life? Did they move around much? How was school, both academically and in terms of friendships? What is their work history? Information about relationships is relevant here – friendships, partnerships or marriage. Does the client have children and if so is additional support needed for their care?

A brief but systematic review can help set the context and sometimes reduce anxiety and distress, as it distracts from current concerns. Sometimes the number of events that have influenced the client's current state may be extensive and not appreciated by the client – so they blame themselves for not coping at a time when they have a 'right' to feel under stress.

Other areas to consider are current substance misuse and history of it – it is usually important to have details of alcohol consumption or use of illicit drugs. If there is evidence that this may be a problem or has been a significant problem, a full substance misuse history should be taken (see Chapter 6). Such evidence would include use or suspected use of illicit drugs or alcohol intake over recommended levels. (Such guidelines have varied over time and with the agencies making recommendations but, in this context, a maximum for men would be three units a day (average); and for women, two units a day). A misuse history should also be taken if there are concerns about the effects of alcohol use (e.g. binge drinking, craving a drink, guilt about drinking or using alcohol to relieve withdrawal symptoms).

A forensic history also needs to be considered. Asking about any criminal convictions can be provocative or reinforce depressive feelings of guilt and needs to be handled carefully. Where aggressive behaviour or manner doesn't appear to be a feature, discussion of contacts with the police may not be relevant, but where there is any doubt, gentle enquiry is important for risk assessment. The evidence seems to be that clients tend to be relatively honest about convictions but nevertheless some may not disclose them where they exist or may minimise them. Subsequent questioning and further investigation may then be necessary. Impending court appearances may be very relevant to presentation as a stressor in their own right. The client may also consider that a psychiatric report would be advantageous in mitigation or sometimes to avoid or postpone a court appearance.

Discussion of social interactions often provides a picture of the client's ways of relating to others (essentially their pre-morbid personality; what they were like before becoming ill), and can again be valuable in terms of knowing what they are usually like and the sort of interests and activities they involve themselves in.

Family, friends, money and home – the current social system

We discussed briefly in the section on preparing for assessment how somebody's intimate social system (friends, family, place of residence) can be both a source of stress to trigger crisis and a source of support to resolve it. So questions need to be asked about the client's domestic situation *without assumptions*. In the client's individual assessment, they may have shared information about family and relationship history. By looking at who is there for the client now you are assisting them in identifying potential sources of support, which means the assessment is useful to the client as well as to you. It has been an intervention in its own right. The presence of a spouse at home does not necessarily reduce risk: we need to ask about the quality of the relationship. Marital discord or domestic violence are often triggers in crises although many more husbands, wives and partners give hours of care and attention to their partners at great emotional cost to themselves. We need to know who is at home, how old they are and how the client relates to those around them.

For people living either alone or with friends, there are other issues. Depending on how much the client wishes to share with friends, it can be an extra stress for a house-sharing client to mask their mental health crisis. The same questions need asking – who are the people who matter in your life and how are they? A precipitating factor in the crisis could be a mother's illness while support could come from a neighbour to some measure in practical and even emotional terms.

Of course the person who causes stress to your client could be the same person who is willing to offer support. For example, the behaviour of a family member who drinks heavily could lead to repeat depressive crisis presentations for a mental health client, but it could be that family member who will assist in safety planning by monitoring medication and staying up all night with the client. In these sorts of cases, the most effective crisis prevention strategy is a family intervention. At assessment stage you just have to live with the conflicting dynamic, while ensuring that safety comes first (e.g. by referral to organisations for those experiencing domestic violence like Women's Aid).

Money troubles are a cause of marital arguments and money can be a large factor in family disputes and stress as well as for individuals. Some people are more at ease discussing financial problems than others. For some it can be hugely embarrassing but specific questioning may allow them to disclose such issues. The reasons for the difficulties are worth eliciting if they are agreeable to this. There are a range of possible reasons, from a change in social circumstances (e.g. being made redundant), to difficulties in managing finances, often through the effects of the mental health problem (e.g. depression), to excessive spending as a result of mania, substance misuse or gambling. Gathering information, even in the crisis, can allow a way of managing the problem to be drawn up.

Housing is an interesting part of assessment that was previously seen as the sole domain of social services. Questions about housing include whether the client has somewhere to live, whether it is of a reasonable standard and whether there are rent or mortgage arrears. Practical issues are important but including housing in assessing somebody's domestic support system is also about acknowledging what where somebody lives means to them. It is the difference between assessing 'home' and 'housing'. For some people their home is a place of refuge, where they feel safe. A threat to this is sufficient to cause a crisis (e.g. letters about arrears or fear of loss of the home through divorce proceedings). It can also be easier to sort out home support for acute mental health distress when the client has a home that feels comfortable to them.

Conversely, for many clients, home is never a particularly cosy place. This may be to do with lack of space if a family is large, may be connected with sad memories, or as a result of external community-based stressors such as neighbourhood noise levels, harassment and vandalism. Either way, we spend a large proportion of our time in the four walls we inhabit and this strongly influences our mental health. The worst-case scenario is when the client is homeless, in which case finding them a roof has to be the first focus for intervention.

Neighbourhood and occupation – the community system

We looked at general community mapping or profiling earlier on in the chapter. Whatever your own knowledge of the area it is valuable to get the client's view of their neighbourhood. Some people are oblivious to blatant drug-dealing in their street while others are devastated by mere rumours that it goes on. In rural areas there may be issues of isolation and lack of amenities and transport. For some people who may be fearful of using local shops or of going out in the dark, it can be helpful to support them to identify positives about their communities – the supports as well as the stressors – and this is the case wherever people live. They may feel resigned to accept their habitat rather than looking at what they like and value or what upsets them about it.

Occupation is a major part of any assessment. How does the client spend their time and do they enjoy or value what they do? As with any other part of the system, work can be a stressor. There may be issues concerning workplace bullying, occupational stress, monotony, redundancy or disciplinary procedures that impact on a client's mental health. For some people, being in meaningful employment is a protective factor for reasons of self-esteem, socialisation and, if in paid work, increased financial security.

Work within the home as a parent is as exacting a job as external employment with much longer hours and no annual leave. We have in the past come across a doctor's letter referring to 'this unemployed woman who has three children', which would be amusing if it wasn't a glaring statement about the low social value society usually places on being the carer of children. Clients in this situation tend to be women. We have noticed anecdotally that the male carers of children are more likely to be praised for taking on what may still be seen as women's work. There is a need to be aware that if a client sees their role in life as insignificant or as a failure, this may not be about individual pathology but about the internalisation of negative ideas considered to be acceptable in the wider social arena.

This issue brings us to the fourth dimension of the client's system that impacts on their crisis.

The political environment

Whether you choose to call a mother 'unemployed', a 'housewife' or 'a parent working at looking after her kids' is a political decision. The assumptions and values that surround us permeate our work without us often questioning them. The risk of not questioning so-called 'given' values is that the oppression that lies within those values goes unchallenged and can be perpetuated into the mental health assessment and subsequent interventions.

On most generic mental health assessment forms there is a section in which to write about 'diversity' or 'culture'. This tends to be used to state the client's religion or ethnicity. In fact it is much broader than that. It is an invitation to look at the variety of ways in which the client might experience harassment, discrimination and social exclusion. Over time, the groups of people who are vilified the most in our society tend to change depending on the politics of the period. At various times in recent years, lone parents have been the trendy social evil, and young people have been demonised for being potential criminals. Currently the favourite enemy is the asylum seeker, particularly if there is any possibility that they are an 'economic migrant' rather than a torture victim. Putting aside the range of oppressive regimes around the world that people rightly deserve sanctuary from, we have rather short memories in being so stressed about economic migration. Most industrialised countries including our own have had their wealth built on the basis of economic migration, from within the country's borders, or as now, within the European Union, and from without. If any of us were very poor and couldn't support our families, it would be pretty rational to try and cross borders to find work. However, to be an 'economic migrant' is a term of abuse now, used to justify making vulnerable, isolated people feel unwelcome, to harass them or else in some cases to justify horrendous and even fatal racial attacks.

Some groups facing prejudice have paper protection but they are still vulnerable to assumptions being made about them, to facing discrimination or verbal or physical assault. The word 'gay' is now a term of generic abuse for schoolchildren meaning something is no good or rubbish. Black people are still more likely than white people to be stopped by the police, be unemployed, if male, imprisoned or excluded from school. Overall, inpatients from the black Caribbean, black African and other black groups are more likely (by 33 to 44 per cent) to be detained under the Mental Health Act 1983 when compared to the average for all inpatients.[8] They are also less likely to be offered psychotherapy and more likely to be given extra-high doses of medication.[9]

So your client could be facing oppression from all sorts of angles. We know that the rates of severe mental illness are high in urban areas of high social deprivation. This is not primarily because people with severe mental health problems are impoverished by their mental health and end up moving to such areas, though there is some gravitation of people with mental illness and substance abuse co-morbidity towards those areas where there are hostels and services for the homeless community. By and large, however, it is the experience of being in an urban environment of poor housing, high crime rates and poor facilities that can contribute to mental health difficulties.

Awareness of this can help on two levels. It helps the individual to acknowledge any stress they feel from their environment and militates against self-blame. A tendency has been described for professionals to 'seek psychological explanations for events rather than to explore complex interactions between the social and psychological dimensions of problems'.[10] If practitioners can take a more person-in-system approach to assessment then it is a move towards a more multi-dimensional awareness of the client's experience. Sharing an assessment that takes a truly psychosocial approach means people are less likely to be blamed (or feel blamed) for their mental health problems.

Awareness of environmental factors can also lead to more useful plans of intervention that may include a housing move or support from a community group. The assessment is also useful on a structural level. When a client presents in crisis, an individual plan of support is drawn up. However, when a number of people present from a particular area, awareness of locality issues can inform service development to make sure that community needs are met in the future.

Helping your client to name areas in which they may feel oppressed or undervalued can work against self-blame. To work in an anti-oppressive way, the client's experience has to be validated by the professional listening. If, as professionals, we do not know or understand the client's perspective, it is fine to say so, listen and *learn*.

Additional aspects of assessment

We have given a broad overview of a mental health assessment interview but there are further aspects of individual assessment which are necessary when seeing clients in a mental health crisis. The first is the mental health examination. It provides a way of guaranteeing thoroughness and standardisation in assessment. Instead of relying on 'gut feelings' that the person is depressed or obsessional, it ensures that the relevant features (e.g. not just what is said but how it is said) are noted. The second is the issue of physical health problems, as these are important in their own right, are often neglected and misinterpretations of symptoms can occur when clients present in crisis.

Assessing mental state

What people say is an essential part of any assessment. However, what you observe about how a client presents and appears is also very important. The 'mental state examination' has been developed for this purpose and while it is used more by psychiatrists than other team members it is increasingly being incorporated in generic team assessments. How clients present is often taken account of intuitively, but formally considering it has the advantage of ensuring that it is systematically appreciated and reduces the potential for bias. Defining exactly why we think someone is depressed can be crucial in some circumstances. For example, someone may say they are not depressed but their non-verbal communication suggests otherwise and alerts you to caution. Conversely, someone from a different cultural background may be perceived as hostile when they are simply expressing themselves forcefully, and there are no other indicators of aggression.

Mental state examination is basically a way of describing appearance, mood, behaviour, thoughts, insight and cognitive function. It is very important to stress that these descriptions should not be judgemental but informative and contribute to an overall assessment. Being specific in descriptions and recording verbatim statements about thoughts and mood can be very valuable as, although they may not be understandable immediately, they may later become clearer and what seem to be delusional thoughts or strange behaviour or appearance may begin to make sense. You should consider the following:

- *Appearance*. Does the client appear as you'd expect? Are they casually or formally dressed with good eye-to-eye contact or does their appearance seem neglected or strange in some way (e.g. wearing shorts when it is snowing)? Neglect may be caused by depression or poverty; strange appearance can result from mania or be 'in the eye of the beholder'. However, these influences are present in any assessment and acknowledging them and using them appropriately is very important. If your perceptions are biased by racial, gender or other stereotypes, systematically examining appearance and other areas of the mental state can be helpful in exposing this.
- *Mood*. How do they describe subjectively how they feel? They may describe being anxious; is how they look consistent with this? They may say they feel fine but look very depressed or suspicious, which will be worth following up.
- *Behaviour*. Is there anything unusual about it? Is the client overactive, angry, slowed up? Are they distracted? Are they looking around without there seeming to be a stimulus for it? It may be that they are hearing voices or that they are hyper-vigilant – or that they've got an itchy collar. It is important to ask further about causes for any behaviour that is unexplained.
- *Thoughts*. Enquiring about suicidal thoughts is mandatory in crisis assessments but there are other thoughts that are relevant such as hearing voices, experiencing paranoia, guilt, fear, anger or obsessional thoughts. Thought disorders include abnormalities of:

  o flow of thought – expressing themselves slowly or rapidly;
  o stream of thought – derailment (where there seems little or no connection between thoughts expressed), 'knights-move' thinking (where the link can be spotted but seems tenuous), etc.;
  o possession of thought – withdrawal or insertion, thinking people can read their thoughts or take them away or put thoughts in their mind;
  o content of thought (e.g. guilt, suicide, obsessions).

- *Insight*. What do they think is wrong with them? Do they think they need help? Blanket statements about poor or 'lacking' insight are not very helpful. You may not be able to agree with the client about diagnosis or that they are ill but they might still be quite prepared to accept help in the form of medication or social support.

- *Cognitive functioning.* Assessment of cognitive functioning occurs as the overall assessment progresses and need not be systematically assessed if communication is satisfactory, memory for past and recent events occurs and orientation in time and place is undisturbed – i.e. knowing where they are and when it is. If there is doubt about this, especially suspicion that a neurological illness such as dementia is present, assessment using a proforma such as the Mini Mental State examination is worth considering. Otherwise, in crisis, there is rarely a case for formal cognitive testing lasting more than a very brief period as it can be obstructive to dealing with the client's distress and developing an effective relationship and crisis plan. Formal testing is likely to be much more reliable when the client is more relaxed and past the crisis. Other states that can impede doing cognitive testing include active substance misuse and abnormality of consciousness (e.g. drowsiness).

Where learning disability becomes apparent, specific considerations need to be made in assessing and performing a mental state examination. The degree of disability may have an influence on assessment of psychosis as the client may be more concrete in their statements and more impressionable.

Assessment of physical health

Physical health problems can readily present as mental health crises and need to be recognised and managed correctly. Often a referral will come direct from a GP or hospital and physical screenings have therefore occurred already. However, it can be dangerous to assume this as such screening may have been cursory or the presentation of symptoms or signs may have developed later. People presenting with mental health problems or with a known past history of them are more likely to have physical illnesses than the general population, but may be less likely to have them adequately assessed and investigated in primary or general hospital care.

How then, if you are not a doctor, do you decide whether a medical assessment is necessary, or if you are one, that further medical intervention is warranted? The nature of the symptoms and signs is important. How long have they been present? Where are they located? What physical signs are there? Is the client in pain? Are they breathless? Past history of similar symptoms and association with previous physical illness is relevant. Physical examination therefore needs to be considered in clients:

- newly presenting to a service;
- with a previous physical disorder;
- who are elderly;

- who have suspected or definite abnormalities of cognitive functioning;
- who have physical symptoms and signs (e.g. alteration in consciousness);
- who are admitted to hospital.

Discussion should occur with a medical member of the team or GP for advice if there are any doubts. Nurse-led services in primary care may also be able to advise by telephone or drop-in (e.g. NHS Direct and NHS Walk-in Centres). Physical examination by a doctor may be necessary and they can determine whether this is the case and make arrangements for it to occur.

Even where physical symptoms are not the direct cause of the crisis, longer-term physical illness and disability are important to recognise in themselves and because of the effects they can have on mood, self-esteem and abilities to cope.

This look at assessment has aimed to be quite broad and has emphasised social content to counter-balance the way the book is now structured. The focus on risks and then symptom groups in the following chapters takes a very individual and potentially pathologising pathway. By taking a psycho-social approach, the hope is that we can hold these ideas in our minds when we look at the personal crises and experiences clients present with to services.

In summary:

- assessment needs careful planning to include the safety of those involved, the most suitable venue and the feelings of the client;
- consideration should ideally be given to the involvement of carers or advocates in any assessment;
- there are a number of strata to be acknowledged in assessment – *individual* pathology, symptoms, patterns of thinking and recent life events, *familial* circumstances, community or *social* problems and the *political* context.

Specific assessments

Assessing homeless clients

People are homeless for many reasons and the term 'homeless' is not synonymous with living on the street. Some homeless people do sleep rough but many more stay in hostels, night shelters or else move around between friends and relatives without a fixed address of their own. A person can be homeless due to a recent move to an area to find work or due to severe and chronic life problems.

People who are homeless have a higher prevalence of severe mental illness than the general population. Yet 'junior psychiatrists are six times more likely to consider homeless people to be inappropriate for admission to hospital compared to those who have a home'.[11] The issue of stigma and the exclusion of homeless people has also been noted.[12] Homeless people fall into a mythical category of 'the undeserving'. Assumptions can automatically be made that they are abusing substances or involved in crime. Other concerns are that once a homeless client is admitted to a ward, they will be impossible to discharge and a bed be taken up indefinitely. This is often not the case as they will frequently be less demanding in terms of move-on accommodation, accepting open access hostels etc. Paradoxically, homeless people can lose out on access to community services because of structural geographical boundaries, mistaken beliefs that homeless people will not attend services or a lack of creativity and flexibility on the part of professionals in providing services. Homeless people with mental health problems benefit when there is a specialist service that addresses their needs as a distinct group.

In assessing a client presenting with mental health problems, the assessment should follow the same lines as with any other client, so the fact of their homelessness should not obscure the individual's symptoms of mental disorder or psychological distress which need to be validated so that the client can be supported to manage them.

As with all assessments the factors that trigger, maintain or exacerbate poor mental health need to be identified. In this context homelessness and its impact on the client needs to be discussed and understood along with other social issues and personal history which should not be forgotten in the face of a housing problem. Again, general assumptions are of no value. The questions to ask clients about housing are:

- How do they feel about their particular housing situation? For example, some people feel safe in hostel accommodation due to good staff support, company and routine or less restricted by being able to move round. For others homelessness may be a terrifying or very unsettling experience.
- What are the client's goals? Would a client living on the street like help to find a hostel placement, is a place of their own the priority or is company preferred?
- What does the client need or want in order to achieve their goals? For example, help to find a roof, skills to live independently, advocacy and support to deal with housing departments or benefits offices.
- Is the client in urgent need of anything fundamental such as food, shelter or blankets for warmth?

People who are without stable housing can have complex social problems contributing to their mental health difficulties which in turn can be very complex. Multiple diagnoses combine with adverse life events and circumstances creating a spiral of distress, exclusion and disability. They may also have immediate needs which require attention. This means that work with them in a crisis situation can take more time than may be available for the practitioner doing the assessment. In the absence of a specialist homeless health care team, this is where knowing your local services and community is so valuable. The best approach to helping people with these needs is a multi-disciplinary one, involving the community mental health teams, the local authority, housing providers and relevant voluntary services.

Assessment of carers

In the UK, long overdue recognition has recently been given to carers' needs and a statutory basis for this to be addressed established.[13] Carers have the right to an assessment of their own needs when caring for a relative who has an illness or disability such as severe or enduring mental illness. Caring can take many forms and is not always about practical tasks and medication administration. It may be about emotional support or being around in times of crisis to dissuade someone from self-injury.

Most mental health teams now have a system or even a specific worker in place to work with and support carers. They may conduct carers' assessments and organise support groups or information sessions. However, aiming for best practice and because it works towards positive outcomes for the client, it is worth giving thought to how carers are supported while the client is in crisis. The crisis for the client is likely to be distressing for those who care for and about them and mental health professionals should acknowledge this.

We discuss issues of confidentiality in work with carers in Chapter 3. Such issues need to be discussed with the client if they have not invited their carer into the assessment. Once this has been clarified, a line of approach can be discussed with the worker and the client. It is not acceptable to leave the carer not knowing what is going on or who to contact if they need help. Carers need as a minimum:

- To be listened to, whether or not you have permission to discuss anything.
- Information that *can* be given (e.g. a number to ring if the situation deteriorates, an out of hours number, how to contact a doctor and what to ask for depending on the local cover system).
- To be given information about their right to be referred for an assessment and about support groups in the area. This is particularly the case when there are carers involved in carrying out the plan to support their relative in crisis.
- Information about medication changes and likely side-effects.
- To know what the plan of action is, when the next visit will be from services and if a package of care is being considered.

Many carers are with the client 24 hours a day and they are often the person the client talks to if they are bothered by voices, anxiety or suicidal thoughts. Clients may tell their carers things they feel unable to share with a mental health professional for fear of being judged, over-medicated or hospitalised. It is crucial to build a relationship with carers that is distinct from, though linked to, the client–worker relationship. The other practical issue to bear in mind in a crisis is that the carer will be stressed. Carers have been accused of being cross or difficult in a crisis situation. The carer may not have slept for a while and/or may have been passed from pillar to post in their attempt to access help for the client. If this is acknowledged and an apology given if appropriate, communication can be much improved.

There is also the possibility that the crisis may have come about from the carer's own breakdown (a situational crisis, as described in Chapter 1). There may be a health problem for the carer that is quite unrelated to their caring role. However, it may be the case that the carer has been inadequately supported and the stress of caring has become too much.

In these instances alternative care such as respite or agency help may be useful and would involve a client assessment. Yet the most urgent assessment would be a carer's assessment. In discussion with the client and carer a more supportive package can then be drawn up or the client can be supported to do more independently if this is appropriate. The process of being heard can also be hugely beneficial for the carer.

Sometimes the result of a carer's assessment is that no extra services are forthcoming, or services are not available or else not acceptable to the client or other family members. In such cases carers can get enormous support from meeting others in the same situation and from advocacy for themselves in any battles they are having with statutory services. Carers therefore need the number of their local carer group and any local helplines that exist. Useful websites include www.rethink.org; www.carersonline.org.uk; www. mentalhealth.org and www.mind.org.uk.

Young carers

Significant numbers of children and young people provide care for a member of their family. Young carers are not necessarily teenagers; they could still be at primary school. They carry out the same tasks as adult carers and may look after the younger children in the family. They may be administering medication and offering emotional support to a disabled or unwell relative. Like adult carers, they will worry about the person they care for.

Some of these young carers are looking after someone who has a mental health problem. They may assist with practical tasks or looking after younger siblings. They may also offer emotional support, and this can be overlooked when a client's needs are being discussed.

We usually ask the client if they have a carer without defining what that means, and the client may not identify their child as being a carer. Asking broader questions about how the children are and whether they have a carer role can bring useful information to the fore. One child may be 'a great help around the house' while another 'pops out to the shops for me if I am having a bad day'.

Family members being supportive to each other is family life at its best. Every family has times when ill-health strikes and everybody has to pull together. Yet when ill-health becomes severe and chronic it can start to put a strain on caring family members, and young people are particularly vulnerable for the following reasons:

- *Invisibility.* Children are sometimes assumed not to be involved in care-giving and their needs may not be identified. They may be at school when assessments take place so their contributions are excluded. It may be assumed by the professionals that they are too young to have a carer role or the client may feel too embarrassed to mention it, feeling they may have failed in their parental role. Children absent from school are usually assumed to be behaving badly rather than because they are worried about a family member and truancy of a child who could be a carer should be looked at sensitively.
- *Age-appropriate support needs.* Carers need support in order to continue caring, whether they are adults or children. Until recently, because of the assumption that carers were adults, services for carers were geared towards adults. Leaflets about medical conditions were written with adults in mind and carer services in mental health tended to involve groups in the evening or sitting services.
- *Emotional vulnerability.* Young carers are vulnerable emotionally because of their age. One concern is that young people may wrongly believe themselves to be emotionally responsible for somebody they could ordinarily expect to be responsible for them. When children and young people care for adults with a mental health problem they can be in a position that would be challenging for an adult to cope with. For example, a child could find themselves having to advise and guide a parent with mania about what is appropriate behaviour. A child may have to take on responsibility for younger siblings if a parent becomes so unwell they cannot function and there is no other adult support available. There are also times when a child feels they need to hold onto their family member's medication for fear they might overdose and that is too heavy a responsibility to be held by someone under 18.

Most people who suffer with mental health problems will ensure that their children are never put in such a vulnerable position, either by hiding the severity of their symptoms, by enlisting extra adult support in times of crisis or by spending time when well in explaining the nature of their mental health problem to the family and having a plan for everyone to follow in times of relapse. However, professionals should not *assume* that this is what is happening. There are still some professionals who do not 'think family' at assessment, so clients may not get the support they need to organise their loved ones to be able to cope.

The needs of young carers include:

- A right to an assessment of their own needs. This is particularly import-ant for children as they are still developing themselves and their needs should be taking a higher priority than those of adults.[14] The profes-sional carrying out the assessment should be somebody with experience and knowledge of work with children and young people and this may require a different service than that received by adult carers.
- Information about the mental health problem in their family, set out in language that is accessible to them. This can be difficult, though the MIND website (www.youngminds.org.uk/family) has information which is young-people friendly. Young people might also want somebody to talk to in private about their worries and this should come from young carers' services or youth counselling services.
- The need to be involved in the care plan of their family member to a level which is appropriate to their age and understanding. A very young carer can understand the words, 'Dad is feeling poorly and can't do very much at the moment so we are giving him some tablets and we will visit twice a week to help him get better. Mum and dad have told us what a great little helper you have been.' An older child can receive a more sophisticated explanation. As with all conversations with carers, the client needs to give permission and some clients are reluctant to worry their children. This is quite right except when, as is often the case, the children are worried already. Children are not stupid, they are just young. They are quick to pick up on changes in a parent's mood and behaviour and are sometimes aware of parental self-harm and suicide attempts. Even when children do not take on a carer role, it is a good idea for parents to talk to them about the mental health problem so that they can share their own anxieties and receive the essential reassurance they need that it is not their fault and not their responsibility.
- A childhood. Children and young people need the chance to be precisely that, children and young people. They need time away from worry and responsibility to have fun and play. Many services for young carers have been set up to do that, taking children out at weekends to just enjoy themselves. It is a service very much welcomed by clients as well, who can take pleasure from seeing their children being carefree and their extra contribution to the family being acknowledged and rewarded. See also www.youngcarers.net and www.childrenssociety.org.uk/youngcarers.

When English is not the first language

There are times when the person to be assessed does not use English as their first language and the assessment has to take place via an interpreter. This may not necessarily be for the client: the carer or other family members may be the people who need this service.

In deciding whether an interpreter is necessary, the referrer will often provide guidance. However, it is often best to ask the client or the family directly about their language of preference, possibly by telephone before the assessment. It is worth being mindful that stress can affect an individual's grasp of a language that is not the one which they use to think. So a client who speaks English fluently in a GPs surgery may struggle more when in a mental health crisis. It is always better to err on the side of caution and have an interpreter that is not strictly needed than to miss crucial information through language difficulty or misunderstanding.

Interpreting services

Most urban areas have well-run interpreting services which use trained, highly skilled interpreters used to working within the boundaries of confidentiality. Good interpreters can often alert professionals to issues that would otherwise be missed (e.g. that the client is using words in a way which makes no sense in that language and culture or that the person's use of language indicates some learning disability or physical problem). Where such services exist, interpreters can be found speedily enough for crisis assessments. In most areas there is an awareness of the common languages spoken and interpreting provision has been made.

There are times however when there may be a need for an interpreter using a particular language and there is nobody readily available who can help. Local and national community organisations can sometimes assist in these circumstances and the local interpreting services can contact organisations elsewhere for assistance. The problem is that this can take time.

When there is no interpretation service available, there can be a temptation to use a family member or friend to assess the client. There are many problems with doing this, the most notable being:

- *Lack of confidentiality* – the friend may go and tell anyone what has taken place and if the client fears this he or she may not give full information.
- *Poor interpreting* – an unofficial interpreter may roughly translate what is said both ways so important information could be lost. An untrained interpreter may also change a client's emphasis.
- *A client may not want the family member or friend to know what is happening* – either because it involves something they are ashamed to share, or they fear disapproval or, more commonly, they do not want the family

member to be worried or upset. This can lead to serious errors in the risk assessment and management plan.

The only way forward when there is a delay in finding an interpreter is to balance the risk of doing nothing against any harm that could arise. The common-sense approach is to do what is necessary with the resources that exist. If a client is at imminent risk, for example standing on a bridge threatening to jump, then any person who can communicate by language or signs should be used. On the same principle, if a person is being left for a long period it is better to get some kind of communication going using anybody available, to reduce the client's distress and isolation and get some idea of what is going on. Getting the client's views on who they might like to translate for them gives them some control over the situation if there is a choice.

Risk should not be used as an excuse not to find an interpreter, and a full and comprehensive assessment should be carried out as soon as the trained interpreter arrives. An alternative in an emergency may be a telephone interpreting service where these are available, which while not ideal, can assist in providing basic information.

If the person is hearing impaired

As with people whose first language is not English, some people who do not hear use sign language and signers can be used as interpreters. Most areas will have a local deaf association that either provides this service or can advise practitioners about where to find an appropriate person. There can be difficulties with assessment when a deaf person does not sign, through choice or through having lost their hearing more recently. If a client lip reads then attention should be given to seating so that the client can see everyone's faces clearly and if there is more than one professional they should not interrupt each other. If a client neither signs nor lip reads then assessment can be done creatively with written notes. Some health venues have a loop system and there may be grounds for moving an assessment to a place where this is accessible.

This chapter now concludes with an assessment checklist followed by a client's view of the assessment system.

Box 2.4 Assessment checklist

Preparation

- Obtain as much information as is reasonable to collect.
- Consider the setting for assessment: risk, appropriateness for client.
- Keep context in mind: social and political.

Assessment areas

- Reasons for referral (from person themselves, carers and referring agent).
- History of the development of these reasons.
- Mental health – history of past contacts for mental health care.
- Risk issues.
- Social circumstances (especially family friends, accommodation, supports and finances).

Mental state examination

- Appearance.
- Mood.
- Thoughts.
- Insight.
- Cognitive functioning.

If possible at crisis interview (if not, needs to be done later)

- Brief personal history:
  - birth and early development – traumatic events;
  - schooling and work history;
  - relationships – friends, sexual partners.
- Family history (especially current situation and relationships):
  - parents, brothers and sisters (relevant others);
  - partner, children – if any;
  - any family experience of mental health problems.
- Substance use (alcohol and illicit drugs).
- Forensic history (contacts with police and courts especially if imminent).
- Physical health (including past and current serious illnesses or accidents):
  - consider need for physical examination.

A client's perspective

Much is written about the power imbalances involved in a mental health assessment, however in my experience little is done to try and address these imbalances. Not all clients are in a powerless situation when being assessed. Assessment relies partly on the client giving correct information and in cases where the client is psychotic and fearful of being admitted, they may be able to 'hold it together' and hide their delusional thoughts long enough for them to go unnoticed. Whereas a client who could be managed effectively in the community but who wishes to be admitted could exaggerate symptoms in order to achieve their preferred outcome from the assessment.

Another point to be raised with regards to a client's powerlessness in a mental health assessment is that as a client, I had enough insight into my difficulties to recognise when I needed intervention and as a result would present to services. I was empowered enough to take responsibility for some of my care and the risk issues associated with my difficulties. This can also lead to difficulties with the respect essential to effective engagement. Experience as a client, carer and professional has highlighted to me the lack of respect from the professional to the client and their family members during assessment. Some professionals, for various reasons, have difficulty in engaging with clients who have good insight into their problems and families who are well-educated in the field of mental health. The need for the client's and their family members' wishes and thoughts to be acknowledged and respected is essential to the engagement process.

Many people in mental health crisis will present at accident and emergency. In the case of self-harm or overdose the client is usually treated by non-mental health staff who are not trained specifically to deal with clients in emotional crisis. As such some staff may show negative attitudes towards the client, believing their behaviour to be manipulative and therefore putting the client off from seeking help in future.

I am in total agreement with the section in this chapter referring to the presence of trainee professionals in assessment. The client should be asked before the assessment takes place and informed that, if they agree to the presence of a trainee, they can ask them to leave at any time.

Community mapping is a useful exercise. It can identify possible sources of support and widen clients' social network. However, community mapping normally focuses on one aspect of the client's life, for example mental health problems, and as such the mapping exercise is already limited. This can then mean that the only places clients are signposted to are projects who work with clients with mental health problems. This can be good and provide the client with a support network who can, in part, have an understanding of the difficulties they face, however, it also adds to the segregation of people with mental health problems from society and therefore increases social exclusion.

Carmel

Chapter 3

Crisis planning

There are certain considerations that are common to intervening in all crisis situations whatever the outcome of the assessment or setting in which it occurs. For individual crises the assessment information needs to be converted into a crisis plan, communicated, taking into account confidentiality considerations, and acted upon. Developing collaboration with crisis planning generally, and specifically (e.g. with the use of medication) also needs to be considered. In this chapter we will also look at situational crises (initially discussed in Chapter 1), when the crisis is occurring *around* the client (e.g. closure of their hostel accommodation) without necessarily being caused by an increase in the severity of their mental health problem.

From assessment to care plan

Assessment will have provided information on which to act. This may be very limited because of circumstances or it may be varied and detailed. Initially we will discuss planning on the basis that a full assessment has been possible and then adapt this for circumstances where information is very limited.

Formulating assessment information into manageable, understandable and communicable shape can be done in a variety of ways. The end product needs to be a plan of action which takes into account assessment information, client wishes and resources available. It may be possible to go straight to a crisis plan without detailed consideration of formulation – certainly without going through the process of developing a written collaborative formulation with the client. But where there are uncertainties the following process may help with understanding and completeness.

Formulation needs to include:

- *Current problems*. A clear statement of what the client describes their current problems as being.
- *Predisposing factors (vulnerabilities)*. What are the important issues that precede the current crisis?

○ Is there a family history of similar problems?
○ Is there a previous personal history of mental or physical health problems?
○ Is there an ongoing mental or physical health issue?
○ Have there been events in earlier life, especially childhood, that are relevant?
○ Is the person living with indicators of high social deprivation, such as poverty, poor housing or high rates of crime?
○ Is the person socially isolated?
○ Are there particular personality vulnerabilities – a pattern of problems coping or relating to others (e.g. through over-dependence, impulsivity or perfectionism, or isolation)?

• *Precipitating factors (triggers)*. What are the triggers to the current crisis? This is not always obvious to the person themselves or to others around them – sometimes it is the accumulation of problems or the 'wearing down' of individuals and carers. There may be a multiplicity of stresses that a person has coped with for years and one extra small issue causes them to collapse under the strain. It may be a problem for others, leading to a reduction in support that is relevant, or it may even be a reminder of previous trauma or other distressing events.

• *Perpetuating factors (maintaining factors)*. These may not be as relevant in an initial crisis but can be important in recurrent crises or in preventing further ones. For example, a carer's coping strategies may be to try to help by doing too much for the client or trying to change their behaviour by criticising them. Any of the triggers that are left unresolved can become perpetuating factors, such as a debt problem, being in an abusive relationship or being constantly subjected to harassment or noise pollution. Perpetuating factors include internal factors such as negative or unhelpful thoughts (e.g. 'I'm useless so there is no point trying' or 'the best way to deal with problems is to ignore them and hope they will go away').

• *Protective factors (strengths)*. These can be individual or environmental. What are the positive elements that the person can bring to managing the crisis (e.g. sociability, intelligence, physical health and creativity)? Environmental strengths include carer support, friendships, availability of community groups, communities of worship such as churches, gurdwaras or the mosque, and a home where the person feels comfortable and safe.

It can be helpful to identify key thoughts, feelings, behaviours, social circumstances and physical symptoms arising from the assessment as this enables each to be directly addressed relating to the key current concerns (such work often forms part of the intervention process described in later chapters). Cognitive behavioural approaches have used this process of formulation in severe mental illness successfully and it can usefully be applied to organise responses to crisis ensuring a broad holistic response. Formulation may just involve drawing the key information from the assessment together with conclusions about next steps. Where there are any complexities, or illustration is needed to convey issues to client or carer (or to assist in discussions with a clinical supervisor) diagrams can be useful (see Figure 3.1 and Appendix 1 for a specimen sheet).

Creating a formulation tool with the client

Some clients and practitioners may find the specimen tool below to be too 'top down' and not sufficiently user centred in its format. It can also be a bit complex and off-putting for people who have literacy difficulties or who lack literacy confidence. It may also exclude people whose first language is not English. If the assessment is being conducted and shared with the help of an

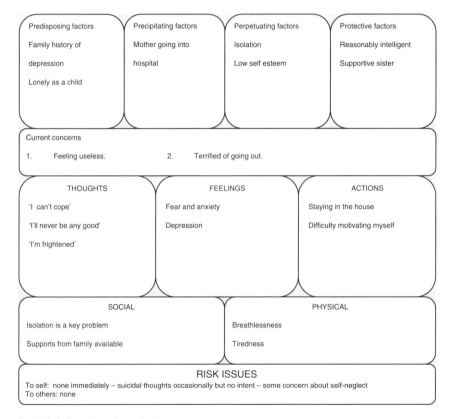

Figure 3.1 Specimen formulation

interpreter a tool in the right language is essential, either as a translation of the one above or as a new tool. The information gathered in an assessment can be presented in other ways, the point being that all relevant aspects of the client's experience are included so the plan is relatively holistic.

Audiotaping can work for some clients who may struggle with the written word through dyslexia or some other reason. Simple diagrams can also be used putting the client's name in the centre of a page with lots of circles around (see Figure 3.2) and a help box with suggestions in it (see Figure 3.3). An advantage of this approach is that it can use colours or pictures so is easier to share with a client if they have literacy or eyesight problems.

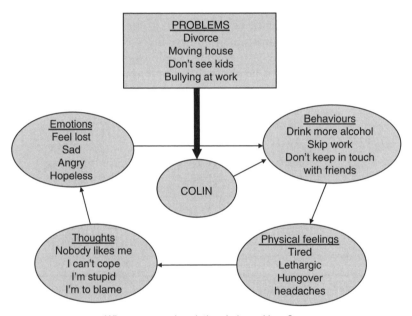

Where can we break the circle and how?

Figure 3.2 Formulation tool

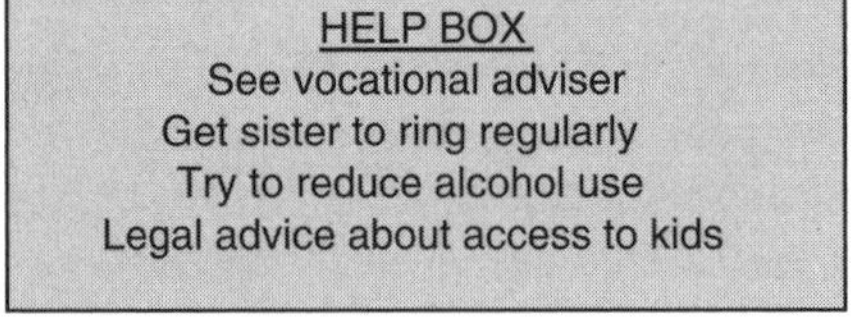

HELP BOX
See vocational adviser
Get sister to ring regularly
Try to reduce alcohol use
Legal advice about access to kids

Figure 3.3 Help box

Immediate decisions following assessment

Following the assessment and formulation, the next decision that needs to be made is whether it is appropriate for mental health services to offer further involvement. The options will be:

- To develop a crisis plan and begin the process of implementing it.
- To discuss whether another area within the mental health service should be asked to offer an assessment and whether this needs to be done urgently or routinely (see Chapter 4).
- To consider whether another service should be involved, e.g.:

  - accident and emergency or other general hospital services for immediate physical health concerns;
  - primary care including any nurse triage systems; where physical or mental health needs may be better met, including primary care counselling;
  - social services, either within the mental health teams or externally depending on the type of social care that is needed;
  - housing department where housing needs predominate;
  - non-statutory sector – counselling is often available through Rape Crisis, young people's services, alcohol or drug agencies, mental health organisations, RELATE (partnership counselling) and citizens' advice bureaus (debt or civil rights issues).

- To discuss whether further involvement of mental health or other services is needed and if it is agreed with client and carer that they are not, discharge. This may need to be discussed with the referrer or at least immediately communicated to them by phone, fax, etc., so that they can respond. If discharge is not agreed with both the client or their carer, the reasons for this difference in views needs to be explored and if discharge does occur, the circumstances discussed in which reassessment would be considered and the ways in which it could be achieved.

Developing a crisis plan

If care is offered, a crisis plan needs to be developed (see Box 3.1).

When it is not an initial crisis the client may have a plan already partly or fully formulated that meets their needs and can be revised in accordance with any new developments. Even if practitioners disagree with the client's formulation or priorities it is consistent with the values of respect, empowerment and self-determination to go along with the client's wishes as far as legally, ethically and practically possible. Sometimes the practitioners may have a different clinical opinion of the best of course of action from those involved initially in drawing up the crisis plan. This may be because different

---

Box 3.1 Crisis plan

A crisis plan will include:

- Individual concerns:
    - mood disturbance (e.g. depression, anxiety);
    - behavioural issues (e.g. self-harm, overactivity, hostility, substance misuse, undereating);
    - thought disruption (e.g. voices, obsessions, delusions);
    - physical symptoms (e.g. pain, over-breathing, confusion).

- Management strategies:
    - Social approaches (e.g. work with relationships, finding meaningful activity, support to the client and family or carers through mental health team, home treatment or admission to hospital – these may be very specific, such as going to the benefit office with a support worker);
    - psychological interventions (e.g. addressing anxiety or voices);
    - biological treatments, especially medication.

- Management of risk issues.
- How to get help? Warning signs of deterioration.
- Who is involved? What are their responsibilities? When are actions to be taken? The role of self-management.
- What needs communicating to others?
- What needs documenting?
- What follow-up arrangements are there?

---

circumstances arise from those envisaged or an alternative treatment approach is thought more likely to be successful However, plans drawn up collaboratively between team and individual client, before a crisis, especially where there has been an extended period of contact between them, need to be given considerable weight in deciding whether to take such alternative courses of action. Discussion will need to take place with the client. Although these plans may not have the power of, say, an advance directive (which in turn is not prescriptive) they are valuable as tools of self-management. One example of this is a Wellness Recovery Action Plan (WRAP), discussed further in Chapter 10. Other examples might include crisis plans drawn up as part of a multi-disciplinary review process or a client's own strong views expressed verbally to friends and carers previously or in the assessment.

Developing a plan from limited information

Judgements about risk and appropriate action are more difficult and need to be more circumspect where information is limited by:

- overwhelming distress;
- thought disorder;
- language difficulties;
- mutism, impaired consciousness or stupor;
- uncooperativeness;
- drug or alcohol intoxication.

Identifying what is not known – areas that need further investigation when possible – is important. Often non-verbal cues from the patient, extrapolation from past behaviour and informant information become important but are inevitably imprecise. Risk assessment needs to take these uncertainties into account, erring on the side of caution, and further assessment may be needed later even using admission to hospital where doubt is sufficient and risk potentially high enough (see Chapter 4).

A crisis plan identifying what immediately needs to happen can still be drawn up but the emphasis will be on trying to develop a collaborative relationship, stabilise the situation and manage risk issues where there is extreme distress. This may include use of medication but not as the only method of achieving these ends. Actions to resolve the triggers to the crisis need to follow. Communication to others, especially the referrer and any carers, either informal or formal, and documentation are very important, while always taking into account issues relating to confidentiality. Details of the assessment and formulation, and of the crisis plan should be communicated along with contact details.

Confidentiality

Confidentiality is a very complex and often confusing area. What is needed for dealing with mental health crises is a sound working knowledge of the principles of confidentiality and how they affect the process of assessment and intervention. Also needed is knowledge of the legal issues concerning capacity and mental health legislation as this affects decisions about the sharing of information in some circumstances.

When practitioners hold in their minds the 'why' of confidentiality, they are bound to be closer to acting ethically. A mental health practitioner is likely to hear information about a client that is intensely personal – about their present situation and also about past traumas. Information given by the client belongs to the client and should therefore be treated with respect. How far it is shared should be the client's choice, with rare contingency arrangements to do with the welfare of the client and other people and certain legal obligations to share.

Rules regarding confidentiality differ for crises where the assessment takes place under mental health legislation. This is because there are certain obligations placed on practitioners acting under various legislations to consult with and/or inform certain relatives, and we will examine these later. For all other crises where the client has capacity, the rules of thumb are relatively straightforward. Every client is assumed to have capacity unless demonstrated otherwise.

It is the client's right to have information about them kept within the health care team. Where a client is routinely referred to services, information about confidentiality should be made available to them and they should know what this actually entails. A number of people may have access to information about the client – doctors, nurses, social workers, administration staff and managers. The client is asked to take on trust that all these people will treat this information professionally and with sensitivity and not disclose it when outside the workplace. In crisis situations, detailed explanations about confidentiality may not be possible or appropriate but simple statements and responses to enquiries about confidentiality need to be made. In general, clients expect what is said to a social or health care worker to be kept within the health care system but if the client seems not to be aware of this or there is doubt for any other reason it may be worth reiterating it. This is especially the case where someone seems reluctant to disclose information as confidentiality concerns may be a contributing factor.

Clients should also know what the exclusions are. If a client suffers or causes those around them to suffer significant harm, there is no option for professionals but to work out who needs to know what for safety purposes (e.g. children's services may need to be told if there is any concern for children's welfare). They need to inform the client of this, except in those rare cases when to tell the client would immediately increase the risk, in this example to the children. Clients should ordinarily be told and involved in the process but if they threaten, for example, to take the children away somewhere, there may be consideration given to not telling the client before child care colleagues are alerted. Similarly, informing the client may not occur immediately if they have made serious threats against others which need to be acted upon.

It is also the client's right to agree to information being shared with others. *A confidentiality policy is not a secrecy policy.* A client may want certain information about their situation to be shared with others, for example, with their housing support worker, a friend or some family members. A common misunderstanding about confidentiality is that information should not be given out. The point is that it is the client's *choice* what is given out and who it is given to. Such information can be an essential part of mobilising a client's social support system. Sometimes the presence of a mental health worker can alert a family to the gravity of a situation which the client had felt unable to communicate previously. In practical terms, to avoid disagreement at a later date, it is often better to:

- support the client to tell the relevant people themselves;
- get a client's signature to confirm that they wish information to be shared.

Many mental health teams and social service departments have standard 'Permission to Share' information and consent forms which are useful in such circumstances. However, these need updating regularly as people's lives change and their views about who they want to help them can alter radically over time.

For clients who do not wish to have any information shared outside their professional care team, there can be stresses when carers, family or friends wish to be involved. Many carers can feel excluded when professionals use confidentiality to avoid speaking with them. However **confidentiality means not sharing without permission; it does not mean neglecting to listen to the information and concerns expressed by others**. It is quite acceptable to tell a client that you are going to listen to their carer's views but you will not be disclosing personal information. It is also acceptable to tell carers you are unable to share information but are happy to hear their views and worries. In fact, what carers overwhelmingly want is advice – 'What can I do to help?' is a frequently-asked question, as are questions about what to do in response to certain changes in the client's behaviour. Practitioners can agree a line to take with the client beforehand or, even better, bring client and carer together so a plan of support can be openly discussed. General advice can be given such as that found in any carer guide to helping someone with a mental health problem, or on relevant websites.[1]

There are times when a client may be assessed as lacking capacity to make their own decision about whether information should be shared. Where a person is assessed as lacking sufficient capacity to make a reasoned decision about who is told about their crisis, the first question to ask is whether the client has an advance directive in place. Alternatively, the client may have written and signed up to something less formal, such as a crisis plan as part of the multi-disciplinary review process or WRAP (see Chapter 10). If a person loses capacity then it is congruent with the principle of respecting information that was discussed earlier to go along with their recorded wishes in so far as this is ethically and legally possible and to act in their best interests.

If somebody has no such plan or is a first presentation, a decision has to be made about who needs to know what. There are probably good grounds for giving the carers general information about responding to the symptoms that the client has disclosed, particularly if they are helping in any treatment plan. Professional carers will also usually be bound by confidentiality, whereas family are not but, of necessity, they need to know about what to do and why.

For example, if a client is so depressed they are barely communicating and not taking fluids and food, his or her family will need to be told of the need for the client to have fluids to prevent the life-threatening risks of dehydration and be given advice on the administration of medication. A discussion will need to take place with the family about whether this can be achieved in the family home and if so what professional input they will need. They may also need to be told at what stage a hospital admission may become necessary. Key people need to know certain information to protect the client's welfare and this needs to be taken into account in relation to confidentiality constraints. Understanding the effects of these constraints on the support that can be offered will often lead to an acceptance by the client of the need to provide relevant information.

When assessments take place under mental health legislation in the UK at present, the practitioner coordinating the assessment has certain obligations. Legislation usually obliges the practitioner to take into account the views of relevant relatives.[2] While this implies listening to the views of those relatives, the very fact that you have contacted them as a nearest relative is giving away the fact that assessment under mental health legislation is taking place, whether or not the client has consented to them knowing this.

Where clients specifically do not want relatives to be contacted there have been difficulties in the past if this clashes with the requirements of legislation. Clients may have relatives who have abused them previously and the need for background information for an assessment could be immensely traumatising if it involves discussing the situation with such a relative. The ratification of the European Convention on Human Rights in many European countries has been helpful in obliging countries with conflicting legislation to develop processes that respect a client's choice about who should be contacted in their family when compulsory admission is being considered. In particular Article 8 about the right to privacy and family life is relevant. Mental health legislation needs to encapsulate the need for carers and family to be consulted about compulsory admissions but to give as much control as possible back to the client as to who the relevant people to consult may be.

Collaboration with crisis planning

If a plan is to be fully effective, the client needs to have cooperated as fully as they are able in drawing it up. However, it may still be possible to work with partial collaboration. There may be specific areas where agreement is difficult and this can involve everything from use of illicit drugs and alcohol, to choice of accommodation, to day activities, psychological therapies and medication. Although the focus is often on medication and substance use, it can be equally or more important to negotiate in relation to other issues. Even when this eventually involves involuntary treatment or admission to hospital, negotiation can still minimise short-term conflict and enhance future cooperation.

Terms used in this context include compliance, adherence, concordance and collaboration. The use of these terms can signify the attitude of the mental health practitioners involved and can easily, if inadvertently, convey to the client an authoritarian stance. Compliance is doing what you are told to do; even adherence involves sticking to a prepared plan which may have involved little negotiation, and concordance can have similar implications. Collaboration means working together and denotes an attitude and style which involves negotiation over crisis planning and implementation in a holistic manner.

It is very easy to become judgemental and confrontational when the practitioner strongly believes that a certain course of action is essential for the client's well-being and they disagree in words or actions. An argument involving the practitioner uttering a series of firmly spoken 'shoulds' and 'musts' can then develop. However, these terms tend to be counterproductive and are best avoided. Dogmatic, all-or-nothing stances tend to lead to confrontation and disengagement. Progress is more likely to be made if it is possible for the practitioner to accept that the client is an individual who, at least in the long-term, will make their own choices. But they might be helped to do so by provision of relevant and balanced information and assistance in weighing up the positives and negatives of the alternatives facing them (i.e. by using an empowering motivational interviewing approach).

Initially listening to and understanding the client's views about a choice engages them and provides material to discuss. In particular, eliciting information which may seem to support not taking medication or using drugs or alcohol can identify reasons which may be very important, and very understandable, in taking these options. The next step may be to rehearse the reasons why medication may be helpful or substances not, with the client taking the lead. It is then possible to discuss the specific issues raised. Often there are ways that can be explored of managing the use of medication, illegal drugs and alcohol, such as:

- If drugs or alcohol are being used to manage voices, anxiety and/or depression, looking at alternatives (see Chapters 6 and 7) and finding out if exploring these options would be acceptable.
- Concerns about side-effects of medication can be discussed and medication tailored to minimise them.
- The problem may be a general dislike of medication and a wish for autonomy from it. Sometimes discussion of this can use analogies with use of medication for physical illnesses. Discussion of the use of anti-hypertensives (for hypertension), hypoglycaemics (for diabetes) and even antihistamines (for hayfever) or medication for migraine can 'normalise' use of medication generally.
- It is also possible to negotiate usage of medication, for example:

- ○   suggest a trial of medication for a defined period with a specific outcome in mind, or alternatively to see if side-effects can be minimised;
- ○   describe the various alternatives available by name and the effects and side-effects of each so that the client can make a choice, providing further guidance (including written information where it may be helpful) and further advice as requested;
- ○   provide advice on dosage and then negotiate; although this may mean that dosages are lower than advisable or medication is used in a less effective, targeted way initially (i.e. only when the client experiences certain symptoms), the compromise reached is more likely to be followed consistently and the mutual respect engendered means that your advice will be respected in the future.

Be ready to adjust your advice to what the client's experience is with medication and substance use. They may have had very negative or positive or equivocal effects and their description of these deserves respect even when it does not seem to comply with standard teaching:

- Some clients do not respond to medication – around a quarter to a third in most research studies with both antidepressant and antipsychotic drugs. There is little to indicate who will respond or not but individual experience may be a guide. Achieving partial response may also be worth discussing as a goal.
- Use of illegal drugs can be complicated Although cannabis is generally believed to aggravate, even precipitate, psychosis in some clients – as seems to occur in the general population – it can relax and be a factor in socialisation. (Cannabis does, of course, have other potential side effects such as those on brain function and motivation, and it is a potential carcinogen.) For other drugs, such as amphetamines, ecstasy and heroin, the argument against use for most clients is stronger but nevertheless understanding why they take them can help address these issues. If all their friends are using illegal drugs, developing other social outlets will be very important and movement to do so may be gradual.

Immediate use of medication or abstinence from drugs or alcohol is often not absolutely essential even following a crisis and it may be better to provide information, verbal and written, and then ask the client to give it some thought and meet later. This can help in not closing off an option totally and sometimes to avoid the need for involuntary measures which can have a negative long-term effect. It is always worth bearing in mind that most mental health problems presenting to mental health teams are likely to require long-term planning and support which can be sabotaged by hasty and ill advised coercive short-term actions.

Where collaboration is not possible

Collaboration is not always possible in a crisis and when this happens, documenting the nature of the disagreement and any advice or warnings given is important. Respect for the client's autonomy and right to make decisions is important and it may be possible to continue to work at some level together or at a later stage. However, there is a duty of care on the practitioner to consider issues regarding the capacity of the client to make decisions and consider whether measures are necessary in the interests of the client's health and that of others.

Assessing capacity

If any doubts arise about the client's capacity to make decisions, assessment of this needs to be made and there are specific guidelines for doing so.[3]

A person is defined as unable to make a decision for himself or herself if he or she is unable:

- to understand the information relevant to the decision;
- to retain that information;
- to use or weigh that information as part of the process of making the decision;
- to communicate his or her decision (whether by talking, using sign language or any other means).

A person lacks capacity if he or she is unable to make a decision for him- or herself in relation to the matter at hand because of an impairment of, or a disturbance in the functioning of, the mind or brain. It does not matter whether the impairment or disturbance is permanent or temporary and any question of whether a person lacks capacity is decided on the balance of probabilities. Although the definition appears very clear, in practice it is rarely 'cut and dried', which is why it remains a clinical decision as to whether the person on balance has or has not the capacity to make the decision under consideration.

There are a number of things to consider:

- a person must be assumed to have capacity unless it is established that he or she lacks it;
- a person is not to be treated as unable to make a decision unless all practicable steps to help him or her to do so have been taken without success;
- a person is not to be treated as unable to make a decision merely because he or she makes an unwise decision;
- an act done, or decision made for or on behalf of a person who lacks capacity must be done, or made, in his or her best interests;

- before the act is done, or the decision is made, regard must be given to whether the purpose for which it is needed can be as effectively achieved in a way that is less restrictive of the person's rights and freedom of action.

The relationship between mental capacity and mental health legislation is currently unclear but it is generally agreed that, rightly or wrongly, there are circumstances where someone may be judged to have capacity to make decisions and yet still be made subject to mental health legislation. When there are significant risks of serious harm to the individual or to others, the use of compulsion as a last resort can become necessary. In these circumstances – especially where hospitalisation or medication or other physical treatments are involved, whether or not the client has capacity – doctors and other specified professionals who can invoke involuntary measures are required to make an assessment. Mental health legislation allows for such intervention but varies in its details in different countries with guidance usually available in codes of practice. General principles apply in relation to involuntary treatment and detention relevant to crisis situations, which involve ensuring that the client meets criteria for mental disorder (or requires assessment for it as it is reasonable to believe that they may), that they are at significant risk of serious harm to self or others and that no alternative is available to involuntary measures (however there is at time of writing, contrary to the European recommendation, a draft Mental Health Act in the UK which lowers this threshold to 'for the protection of others' with no qualification of significant risk of serious harm and the implications of this may need to be taken into account if enacted). Carefully explaining the reasons why (i.e. the specific risks of not intervening), and 'agreeing to differ' can lead to the client agreeing to cooperate or at least not actively resist the intervention. It can also be very important in long-term cooperation. Certain circumstances cause particular difficulties, for example in relation to substance misuse (see Chapter 6) and concurrent physical illness (see Chapter 8).

Situational presentations

Most crises have triggers and clients can often track back their increasing distress to an event or a series of events, or to memories that have been revived without the client having the internal coping resources to deal with the feelings aroused. However, there can be crises when the client may not be suffering any increase in mental health symptoms but an urgent response is needed from services nonetheless. Some examples of such crises might be:

- the death or serious illness of a carer of a client who needs a lot of support when there is no obvious person to take over from within the family, or the family is too grief-stricken to make plans at this early stage;

- a client is facing imminent eviction from his or her home when care is needed;
- a fire in a residential home or a home closure leads to lots of people needing to be quickly rehoused;
- a major disaster at a local airport or train station, as mental health teams contribute to multi-agency crisis response teams for staff support and debriefing, if appropriate (obviously individual presentations will also occur consequent to these events);
- a mental health client has developed a physical illness or has had an accident which leaves them unable to access their usual care and means they have overlapping needs.

Such situations can almost be seen as crises of care or of resources. Even if they are not suffering mental health symptoms, any of the above scenarios or other 'life being turned upside down' kinds of experiences are going to throw the client into disequilibrium. Clients, like any of us, are going to need sensitive support to come to terms with the changes, find a way to manage feelings about losses and move on to a new 'reintegrative' state.

The risk with such crises is that they become a crisis for the organisation with the duty of care, rather than a crisis for the client. This is particularly the case if new resources have to be found at speed. It is notoriously difficult to find a new residential mental health placement for one person and to find places for several people is going to cause significant stress to the care coordinators involved. This can lead to the care coordinator becoming the focus rather than the client. The situation is happening to or around the client, yet their views about what should happen, their choices and feelings about loss and change can get lost in the plans and processes that are 'doing for' rather than 'doing with' the client. The chance of this happening is higher the greater the number of clients that are affected by the crisis.

Ultimately, the resolution of a crisis situation lies with the client, and may take time if the person or people concerned are in shock or suffering high distress levels. There may have to be an initial response to provide crisis care (e.g. a temporary placement but assurances given that this is a stop-gap until a collaborative solution can be found). Where there is a potential conflict of priorities between the care coordinator and the client, there may be a case for the use of an advocacy service. If the service providers are then looking at a solution that is easy but does not meet the client's needs then there is a mechanism to ensure the client's voice doesn't get lost. People are very vulnerable in crisis situations and may feel they have to accept solutions offered to them without consultation and then regret it later.

In the scramble to find new care provision, the concept of opportunity in crisis can be lost. With a loss or bereavement the person requires time but in the situation where a move becomes necessary, there can be the possibility of positive change, such as enhancing autonomy while taking new risks. Might the client be interested in independent living with care going in, for example, or would they prefer to try doing things independently that they would not have considered previously?

When larger numbers of people are involved, good managerial organisation is of great importance. Practitioners can then be given tasks in a briefing session. There can be a split between the role of the person who is hunting down urgently-needed resources and another person who is assessing the client's current needs and emotional state and offering human support.

Most health and social care organisations have coordinated plans in place for larger-scale catastrophes or serious incidents that happen in their area. These cover large accidents with many casualties, tragedies that may occur in the community such as a death in a local school or a particularly horrific crime that affects a great many people. These sorts of crises are outside of the remit of this book as they do not involve mental health as a focus (though people traumatised by serious incidents may well need immediate mental health support which may be managed using the principles outlined in Chapter 5 and later support with PTSD if their experiences are too much to easily resolve).

Chapter 4

Risk assessment and management

Risk assessment needs to be put in context. It is not the most important component of care although it is a part of it. Whether harm occurs to an individual is of course very important, but the quality of each individual's life and the human rights of that person and those affected by their actions take precedence. This is not to deny the importance of reducing harm to self or others but to ensure that an appropriate balance between someone's autonomy, their rights and the rights of others is kept.

In practice, if our focus is exclusively on risk or unduly concentrated upon it, engagement with the person concerned can fail to develop or be damaged. They can feel stigmatised and developing a trusting and confiding relationship can be very difficult. Even where risk seems to be the presenting problem, gaining an understanding of the breadth of the person's experiences and circumstances is not only the most appropriate way to work with them but also helps to assess and manage any risk issues.

So engagement is very important, as is making as full an assessment as practical. Managing crises involves immediate attention to safety issues where there is serious risk of harm to self or others, but once the situation is stabilised, then a fuller discussion and assessment can take place.

In assessing and making decisions about risk, mental health practitioners are often at their most powerful in relation to service users, as they have the ability to recommend or enact compulsory admission and treatment under mental health legislation. Such situations therefore represent a time of high anxiety for clients. It may also be a time of high anxiety for practitioners. This is a matter for concern as it is when assessing risk that practitioners need to be at their most 'cool headed' so that decisions are made with careful consideration and sufficient self-awareness to avoid any premature or discriminatory assumptions. Emotions are expressed differently and more, or less, freely in different cultures and in different families within the same culture, so checking out the difference between perceived risk from high levels of emotional expression and the actual risk based more on present and past behaviour is needed for all risk assessments.

We noted in Chapter 2 that in the UK, black African Caribbean men are far more likely to be detained under mental health legislation than white. However complex the reasons, this phenomenon must be the result of racism, albeit sometimes covert, unrecognised and even unintended at a personal or institutional level. Anybody assessing risk needs to be alert to any prejudices they may hold so that racial and other forms of stereotyping are minimised in decisions made about a crisis plan that manages risk.

There may also be issues about the person presenting late to services or being reluctant to engage because of fear of them, due to their reputation in the community or due to personal experience, or because of difficulties accessing services, perhaps because they are inappropriate or unwelcoming. The benefits of engaging the client in future should not be forgotten in risk assessment.

What this should not mean is inaccurately minimising risk and the avoidance of managing it. As for any client, if a black client needs detention as community support would not prevent, for example, a planned suicide, and the client will not consider voluntary admission, then that person has a right to be detained for their own sake and that of their family and loved ones. What this should mean is that if, as may well happen, that person is angry about being so detained, then judgements about them posing a risk to others should only be made where there is concrete evidence of this.

It is possible to detain somebody with respect, fully explaining the reasons (e.g. that you fear for their safety or health if they remain at home). Their rights of appeal should be explained to them, which can take the heat out of a situation. Admitting professionals can apologise for distress caused and offer to involve family or friends in the admission. This can help to reduce risk to others during the conveyance of the client to hospital and assist with engagement in the future.

Immediate issues

Assessment begins as soon as information is communicated about the need for somebody to be seen and risk issues need to be assessed. Such assessment needs to include information on any actual and potential risks. For all crisis referrals, you would want to know if there was an immediate risk:

- Is the person currently saying they intend to harm themselves or others?
- Are they known to have the means to do so?
    - *Immediately* (e.g. they are standing on the edge of a bridge, carrying a weapon or holding material which can be immediately seriously damaging).
    - *In the near future* (e.g. tablets which can cause significant damage).
    - *Possibly*, because of reports that they have a past history of harm or carrying weapons.

- Are they expressing thoughts of harming self or others but do not intend to do so immediately?
- Who is with them at the moment?

  ○ *Police*: generally, of course, the police will assess and manage risk effectively as they are trained to do, but they may not be aware of all the information available. Also their presence can have a negative impact because the individual perceives threat (e.g. if they have paranoid ideas or previous negative experiences with authorities).

  ○ *Family doctor*: they may have a good relationship which can act as a bridge in engagement with the person. If such a relationship does not exist, nevertheless their interpersonal skills and status can still assist.

  ○ *Family members or other carers*: again a good relationship may help. But where the relationship is ambivalent it can be difficult, especially where the person doesn't want help but carers have called for it. Risk to other family members can be significant and unpredictable. (The needs of children should be taken into account here. They should be protected from physical harm or neglect and from the emotional distress of having to manage distressed or distressing behaviour from an adult carer.)

  ○ *Other mental health worker*: the relationship already established, if any, can be influential but the status of 'mental health worker' may not be positive depending on the individual's perception and prior contact with services.

- Is further support needed?

  ○ *How do you decide?* This will be dependent on the immediate threat to self or others determined by previous known history, current statements and potential to cause harm (e.g. available means). Physical stature may influence this decision but should only be one component in the overall risk assessment.

  ○ *What do those with the person think?* Is the situation calming and stabilising or becoming more difficult?

  ○ *Is it necessary to alert others?* To attend with you, as immediate backup or available if necessary?

  ○ *Who?* Other colleagues including psychiatrists, the individual's care coordinator, or someone who knows the person from the past; relatives; friends; police.

- How much background information do you have?

  ○ From those making the request for assistance.

  ○ From your own past knowledge of the person and the environment they are in.

  ○ From immediately available information (e.g. computer records or crisis warning screens, other professionals and sometimes case records).

Deciding how much time you should spend collecting information can be a difficult judgement. If the risk is immediate and there is danger of harm to the patient or others, calling for support may take precedence. This can always be cancelled if other information is then found, making it unnecessary. Background information can be invaluable: generally the minimum would be to retrieve what is available in the base where you are and supplement it by one or two short telephone calls, or via fax or email if available. This is particularly important from anyone with knowledge of the patient who can alert you to otherwise unidentified risks and also put in context risk information. Waiting for information for more than a few minutes however may leave colleagues and carers unsupported and so it may be appropriate to arrange for information to be forwarded, or assessed and telephoned through.

Risk assessment is a dynamic process which, at best, is an inexact science, involving balancing risks and quality of life, as far as possible, based on the person's own choices.

Risk identification and assessment

You may be going to the person or they may be brought to you. Having the above information will affect your decision about this, i.e. can they be brought safely? Is that appropriate? How much does that inconvenience or even endanger the client and those with them? There are many advantages in going to meet the person when they are in crisis (as discussed in Chapter 2). However, safety should not be compromised unnecessarily.

Should you see the client alone? This was discussed in Chapter 2, but the decision needs to take into account safety aspects. In many crisis situations there are lots of people, from practitioners to concerned neighbours, all milling around. Or the client may be alone. Negative outcomes are reduced and engagement increased by the client having some choice as to who is with them to offer support and by them not being overwhelmed by strange unknown mental health workers.

Securing personal safety and that of others, including the client, needs to be considered. Consider making available an immediate means of making contact for support (e.g. through use of alarms, or if these are not available or likely to be heard, mobile phones). Phones can be set to a specific number so that calling and connection is a one-touch process, with the individual to be contacted made aware of the possibility of such a call and what to do.

Assessing risk with the individual

Assessing risk with the individual should be part of a broad assessment if possible. It is often better to use the general techniques outlined in Chapter 2 to elicit information – allowing the person time to expand on their story of events and then becoming more focused. However, if a client is presenting with statements about risk or harm (e.g. saying that they intend to harm or kill themselves or others), exploring these directly is clearly necessary. This can commence by exploring why they feel this way. How do they intend to do what they are proposing? What might be an alternative – in other words, are there ways of achieving their goals without risk to self or others?

Identify in the assessment:

- *Key individual issues.* This involves assessment of suicidal thoughts, plans and intent to harm self or others with consideration of any actions taken so far. Actions in the distant past or more recently need attention. Did these actions succeed in their objective? If not, why not? For example, where someone has stated that they attempted to commit suicide, what prevented that happening? If they acted themselves to reduce risk (e.g. by calling an ambulance or ensuring that they were found before significant harm had occurred), this will be useful in assessing actual as opposed to expressed intention. However, someone might have changed their mind – their intention – and revert to that same aim later with greater effect.
- *Demographic risk issues* (e.g. gender, age, past history of physical or mental illness).

For assessment of risk of suicidality or harm to others after an act has occurred, ask yourself the following:

- What preparation occurred?
  - Was the act planned in advance?
  - Was action taken anticipating their own death (e.g. settling affairs, writing a will or suicide note)?

- What were the circumstances of the event?
  - Was the patient alone?
  - Was it timed to minimise intervention by others?
  - Were precautions made against recovery or discovery?

- What followed after?
  - Did they seek help to avert the effects of their actions?
  - Did they state a wish to die or harm others?

    ◦   Was their stated expectation that the act would be fatal or specific harm result?

    ◦   Were they sorry that a suicidal act failed or not sorry that an act of harm to others failed?

Consideration needs to be given to relevant areas of risk:

- to self, carers, those cared for (including children and vulnerable adults) and others.
- of harm, death, neglect, exploitation, significant embarrassment (e.g. through disinhibition), distress or disturbance.
- from others (including partners, neighbours, strangers, even mental health services through medication side-effects etc.)

Intent needs to be assessed by finding out about:

- the reasons given for causing harm to self or others;
- the reasons for not causing such harm (e.g. effect on person's own family);
- the stated intention;
- the safeguards in place to prevent serious harm (e.g. knowing someone will be returning at a certain time, using a means not thought to be dangerous, even though it might be);
- religious and other beliefs.

Some situations and circumstances are known to present increased risk:

- when a client stops medication or contact with services if past experience links this with aggressive or suicidal behaviour;
- when a client who has previously offended or attempted suicide under the influence of alcohol or drugs starts drinking again or enters an environment where drugs are commonly available;
- when a client whose aggression to self or others has been apparent in one particular situation (e.g. in the context of a close relationship), enters that situation again;
- anniversaries, annual holidays, and birthdays where these have significance (e.g. in relation to a previous bereavement or relationship breakdown, or to episodes of physical or sexual abuse).

Individual factors to consider include:

- the past history of the client;
- self-reporting by the client at interview;
- observation of their behaviour and mental state;
- discrepancies between what they report and what is observed;

- prediction indicators derived from research (see below);
- implications of positive risk-taking (e.g. voices may be distressing and disturbing but the client prefers to maintain autonomy and not take medication – however the option of medication needs to be readily available without any 'loss of face').

Specific issues about risk to self

Relevant demographic factors from research suggest that suicide risk rises with age (except that it is high in young males). Men are four times more likely to commit suicide than women, and it is highest in divorced men, followed by widows, widowers and those who have never married. It is lowest in married people. Suicide is associated with social isolation, family history, physical and mental health problems, and rates are highest in April, May and June. In people with schizophrenia, increased risk of suicide is associated with previous depressive disorders, previous suicide attempts, drug misuse, agitation or motor restlessness, fear of mental disintegration, poor adherence to treatment and recent loss. Paradoxically (and puzzlingly) however, delusions generally seem not to be associated with increased risk of harm to self and there is reduced risk with hallucinations.[1] There is some contrary evidence that commenting voices with passivity (control override) are a risk factor.

High-risk occupational groups tend to be those who have ready access to means of suicide such as farmers and doctors. Unemployment is a factor and risk is also increased in social class V (unskilled workers) compared to other classes. Suicide attempts raise risk by 100 times in the succeeding year of an episode and risk after discharge from hospital is increased in the first month, especially the first seven days. In depressed patients, factors of relevance include severe dysphoria (persistent low mood), past alcoholism, use of long-term hypnotics and chronic physical illness.

Factors in teenage suicide include hopelessness, running away and 'reckless' behaviour, self-harm and panic symptoms, recent loss and social isolation. A third to a quarter die within two weeks of their birthday. Factors in older people include bereavement and physical illness.

Specific issues about risk to others

Risk factors include a past history of aggression, threats being made towards professionals or others involved in detaining the client, delusions that others are threatening the client's safety, disinhibited behaviour or body language that indicates aggression. Any or all of these indicators do not mean that a client *will* be aggressive. If the police are used to reduce risk, it is vital that they are told why they are there and whether their presence is a precautionary measure or a response to an incident. This should be shared with the client as well so that the situation is not inflamed by police presence. This is particularly the case for those clients who are in the social groups that face prejudice about their assumed potential criminality or aggression, such as young people, black people, or people who have a past police record. Obviously it is always best to avoid using the police if a safe assessment and admission can happen without their help.

At its most extreme, consideration of severe violence is necessary. There have been examinations of homicide cases where people with mental health problems have been involved. These have identified risk factors associated with mental health problems between the ages of 20–40 years in men and women, with twice as many men affected than women. Where mental illness is present, males usually have schizophrenia and females usually have affective psychosis (including puerperal illness). Victims are only very rarely strangers. Co-morbid substance misuse and antisocial personality disorder are important factors.

Combination of risk factors

All factors are, of course, not equal in importance and weighting their influence is a key component of assessment. But how to do this is much less well supported by research. It is in this area that clinical experience is of great importance but there are some obvious issues to prioritise:

- current behaviour indicating intent;
- current statements of intent;
- the seriousness of past actions (especially actual harm to others or the nearness to success of suicide attempts): **'nothing predicts future behaviour like past behaviour'** is an evidence-based statement;
- serious physical and psychological symptoms, especially a combination of them;
- hopelessness;
- a strong family history;
- substance misuse;
- antisocial personality traits.

These then need to be balanced against other factors – it is still possible to have significant risk without any of the above. Combinations of factors would be expected to further increase risk, sometimes exponentially (e.g. previous history of serious assault or suicide attempt, substance misuse and antisocial personality traits).

Risk of neglect

Generally where risk to the client is of neglect, it is family, neighbours or professionals such as police, housing officials or family doctors, who ask for assessment. The person themselves may not have recognised a problem although they may be willing to cooperate. Where this is the case, a crisis doesn't arise – but where the client is unwilling to consider changes to their situation, it can. Assessment of neglect needs to consider what effects this has on the client and on others and how serious these are. The client's wishes and capacity to make decisions need to be considered. Debate and persuasion is reasonable to pursue but where there is limited interference with others or no serious effects on themselves, the client has the capacity to choose and if they wish to continue as they are use of any form of compulsion under mental health legislation is not normally appropriate. It may be that the client's landlord (who may be the local housing department) will take action in relation to the client's tenancy or other measures may be taken if the client is considered a 'public nuisance', but these will be decisions taken at a later stage. Resolution of the crisis may be assisted by setting a time for a case review to be convened so that those concerned can be assured that a review of the situation is to occur. Assessment under mental health legislation may only be made where there are doubts or likelihood that mental disorder is relevant and persuasion unsuccessful. Where others are at risk of neglect, measures will need to be considered to meet their needs. There are some public health measures available (e.g. under the National Assistance Act in England), although they are very rarely used.

Where neglect has become a significant problem, concern about health and hygiene may lead to the client requiring different accommodation. Often this ends up being hospital, because it is simple to access. Where neglect has been long-term, physical intervention may be necessary, especially if dehydration has become an issue, and the need for the client to start taking fluids again is urgent. There may also be a need to encourage clients to eat again at some point but this conversation can be had once engagement is effective. A person's mental and physical health are not separate entities and somebody suffering from undernourishment is not likely to easily regain the energy and motivation that has been sapped by the depression and so this will need to be addressed promptly.

Risk of harm from others

People with mental health problems can be vulnerable to abuse from others. The nature of this abuse can vary from violence to sexual assault or harassment, to bullying or financial exploitation. It may of course be the abuse from others that is causing the mental health problem, such as domestic violence leading to depression, but there are ways in which people with mental health difficulties are additionally at risk.

People with a history of mental health difficulties may fear that they will not be believed if they tell others they are being abused in some way, particularly if they have a psychotic illness or a label of personality disorder.

This fear may be well founded in past experience. Any such concerns raised by clients therefore need to be properly investigated. Clients may also be dependent in some way on the person abusing them, who could be their carer, relative or 'friend'. Clients may fear for their ability to cope if the person is no longer with them or they may not realise the extent of their exploitation – for example, if a 'friend' is stealing money from them. Then there are the instances where clients face harassment for the fact that they have mental health problems, through taunts, threats or even violence, often stemming from misconceptions held by members of the public about mental ill health.

Abuse may take place in a hospital or residential facility where the client is in a relatively powerless situation. Clients may experience a range of oppressive and abusive experiences from other clients or from staff. In addition to the fear of not being believed, clients may be reluctant to disclose what is happening through fear of loss of the service or recriminations from the abuser who could remain in control of the client. If allegations are made against a member of staff, their colleagues may be defensive and reduce support to the client in need.

Adult protection procedures have been established in many services,[2] such as empowerment of clients by making them aware of their rights and of how any complaints and concerns will be dealt with; careful selection of staff, including taking up references and making police checks; and the training of staff to be alert to the possibility of clients being abused or exploited in some way.

When a client tells someone about abuse they are suffering or when a professional develops suspicions that something is amiss, the consequences can be complicated and precipitate a crisis. There may need to be a change of placement for the client despite the fact that they are the wronged person. There may need to be police involvement and clients need support with this and to be protected from recriminations. Difficult issues arise when clients do not wish action to be taken and professionals are concerned about their well-being and safety. The potential conflict between the duty of care of professionals and the client's right to self-determination means that issues of capacity need to be considered along with harm reduction possibilities. These decisions need to fully involve the client and to be multi-disciplinary. It is best to take advice from whoever is taking the lead in adult protection work in all instances when clients may be at risk.

Allegations of abuse by clients have often been dismissed as due to their mental health problems. It is unusual for this to be the case and such allegations need full independent investigation when they initially arise. Detailed accounts need to be taken and it usually becomes clear that there is substance to the complaint. In some circumstances such detail cannot be obtained because of the distress being experienced by the client or because they are simply unable to recall detail – either because of psychological suppression (generally due to the distress entailed in recalling abuse) or memory problems, for example from dementia or head injury. Without detail it may be difficult to proceed, although corroborating evidence may be available or further information emerge at a later stage. Only where detail cannot be obtained and investigated, or where this is contradictory or turns out to be inaccurate, should mental health issues be considered as possible cause. In these circumstances it is often possible to find a connection between the client's beliefs, previous statements and the events described.

The needs and rights of children and young people

Many practitioners still fail to think in terms of family when assessing clients' needs but there has to be an awareness of children and young people's needs when looking at risk management. Parents with mental health problems can and do parent admirably but that should not blind practitioners to any potential concerns about children's welfare, and our clients would not thank us for downplaying these possibilities.

We have already discussed the issue of young carers in Chapter 2, and this is relevant here also. Young people may be acting as carers, holding medication or carrying out adult responsibilities and their views are important, as is the need to provide them with support.

There is an emotional stress on any child or young person when their relative or parent is being assessed and there are perceived risks, even when these do not directly affect the children. Any plan that means the parent is removed to a hospital or to stay with relatives is going to distress children. They will need reassurance and an explanation proportionate to their age about what is going on. If other relatives can give this then that is fine but if they are distressed the mental health practitioner could remind the family and advise them about the children's needs. Where a client is the sole carer of children and has no informal support there may have to be arrangements made for the children to be accommodated by social services if the parent is going to hospital or is too unwell to care for the children. This will cause distress to the whole family. It can be normalised a little by reference to its temporary nature but will still be traumatic for everyone.

Risks to children and young people

Where there has been an emotional risk to children, special consideration of this needs to be part of the risk assessment. Dealing with bizarre, erratic or unusual behaviour can be deeply upsetting for children and young people and they should not be left to manage this alone. Neither should children be holding their parents' medication or taking responsibility above that appropriate to their age. Arrangements need to be made for children to receive explanations and support, again ideally from other trusted family members. If children have witnessed upsetting things, such as a parent trying to self-harm, then they may need additional support and local children and family services may be able to advise families and practitioners on how to access this.

Where there is a physical risk to children, this has to take precedence above everything and arrangements made for their safety. The concerns may be about neglect, not getting fed or young children not being supervised adequately. A child may have been assaulted or there may be a risk of this if a client is lashing out or if the client has strange beliefs and thoughts about the child. If this is the case then the client should not be left where the child is. Children and family social services may need to be called upon for assistance and family members used to provide alternative care for the period of the crisis. Again it may be that social services have to accommodate the children if there is no other family who can help.

The most important message to leave with children in these situations is that none of this is their fault. It is also worth remembering that children suffer from mental health problems too and if they are being adversely affected the family doctor, the school, local support agencies and, if referred to them, local child and adolescent mental health teams may be in a good position to help and advise the family about the support options for stressed and distressed children.

What can you do?

Are the risks such that action is needed:

- *Immediately?*
  - The person is actively trying to leave or self-harm in a dangerous way.
  - Or they have threatened to do so and risk of success is judged to be high.
  - Or despite denying intent to harm they are judged to be at high risk of doing so.
  - The person does not have a carer (including where the relationship is or has broken down) or other protective factors.
- *Urgently?*
  - The person is not at immediate risk.
  - They have carers or others who can be with them.
  - They are prepared to consider treatment options.
- *Routinely?*
  - Risk is not assessed at this time as high (although long-term risk may be elevated).
  - Treatment options are available.

At the scene and on the basis of information so far available:

- Assess the need for instant action. Restraint may seem necessary but should only be considered if sufficient properly trained personnel are available so that this can be done without seriously endangering self or others. The police can be very helpful in these instances.
- In every case, secure the safety of the environment. Prevent access to potential weapons, if necessary removing or deactivating them and ensure that sufficient trained and untrained personnel are present.
- Consider who is with the client:

  - Carers – are there any risks to them now or in the future? Are they going to need emotional support during the process and after it? Is their involvement directly in the assessment likely to make the client feel more supported or less? Are they able to allow the client to tell their own story?
  - The police or other emergency services – what impact might their presence have? Individual police can manage these situations extremely well but occasionally they can increase risk by inexperienced and seemingly unduly forceful handling. It is best to work with them, acknowledging their expertise while contributing your experience in relation to mental health issues. They will generally look to the mental health professionals to lead and advise them except in circumstances where obvious and immediate risk is involved.
  - Children – what do you do if children are with the client? The emotional/psychological and physical risk to them from managing distressed or bizarre adult behaviour needs to be considered. Other family members or child care services may need to be called upon quickly if there is a risk of neglect or physical harm to children.

- Consider if further support is needed. This depends on what the client is saying (e.g. they may need to collect their children from school). How willing are they to engage in safety planning? How readily are they identifying protective factors and showing a willingness to engage with services or informal help?
- If the client wants to leave and there is good reason to be concerned for their or others' safety, try to persuade them to stay at least to be assessed. If they persist in their intention to leave, assess the capability of those present to stop the person leaving and do so if this can be done safely. If not and it is possible and safe to follow them, do so until support arrives. You may be able to continue conversing with them. If this is not possible and they are not already involved, alert the police.

Once a conversation can occur, assess:

- the individual's willingness to remain for further assessment;
- their level of distress;
- their mental capacity to make decisions about their proposed acts;
- risk to themselves and others;
- presence of treatable mental health problems.

If the client has already significantly self-harmed, they will need to be taken for medical and nursing attention to repair lacerations, to reduce impact of medication overdosage or protect against consequences. Speedy responses to overdosage can make a difference. Supportive measures can be used to prevent circulatory or respiratory collapse. When the client's physical state is stabilised, it is important to ensure that risk of further and potentially catastrophic self-harm is minimised.

Where someone has self-harmed, intervention is often not appropriate – at least from mental health services – although brief crisis management may be helpful. These are occasions where self-harm or threat of it has occurred in the context of a relationship problem or life event and either the crisis has led to some form of resolution or the action is now regretted. It may also be that response to such events can be counterproductive.

If the client has not or is not known to have self-harmed, management of risk needs immediate consideration:

- make a full assessment, as above;
- consider what risks exist and how to judge them;
- where significant risks appear to exist or there is doubt, discuss them with another team member or senior practitioner/doctor, if necessary by telephone; this process is valuable in ensuring that the assessment is full and judgement balanced and shared.

A decision needs to be made with the client, carers and colleagues about the effective intervention to manage the risk, taking into account the information gathered. This can be made easier if good crisis plans and documentation of past risk issues and how they were managed exist and are readily available. Once the plan is decided, it needs to be communicated to all concerned: the client, the family or other carers and professionals. Both clients and carers need access to information about how to get help if the situation deteriorates. This usually means emergency telephone numbers for carers or the client. Risk management plans arise from weighing up opposing courses of action. There are risks in allowing somebody to remain at home when they have strong suicidal thoughts. Conversely, there are risks to admitting the client to hospital, such as feelings of failure, risk of assault, loss of social support and status and being less close to caring family members.

Where risk of harm is seen to be relatively low

At the start of the chapter risk management was discussed as being part of a process that is about engagement and assessment. As part of the assessment, the events leading up to the crisis are described and there may be triggers to the crisis identified. If someone is given the chance and the time to express strong feelings, the intent behind what they have said to cause alarm can diminish. A client who has threatened to kill somebody may be able, when given time to talk, to say that they feel hugely angry but can control it. Similarly a client threatening suicide may after discussion be able to reframe their thoughts so that, although they feel like ending it all, they are able to identify reasons not to do so.

The idea of giving *time* is the key here. Many assessments can feel rushed in a crisis with the consequent possibility of missing the chance of letting clients talk themselves out of the crisis. The other advantage of giving time is that a good crisis resolution can help prevent future crisis recurrence.

In situations such as these, the assessment itself is a key part of the intervention. The client and the people who care about them can be offered any of the following to help manage future crises or a flare-up of the current crisis:

* helplines relevant to the client's problem;
* ways to access mental health services locally;
* a jointly-compiled list of strategies to help the client cope;
* anger management techniques;
* relaxation techniques;
* referrals for training in stress management, anxiety or anger management or assertiveness, by services or adult education;
* referral to specific counselling services;
* referral to ongoing help from mental health services if needed or to drug or alcohol services if appropriate;
* family doctor follow-up;
* information about useful, voluntary agencies.

Where risks exist but can be managed in the community

There are a number of variables that can lead to the decision to support somebody at home. Practitioners are inevitably influenced by the availability of resources and support (informal and formal) as well as the cost-benefit of a person being admitted or not. Examples of interventions that can manage the risk in the community include:

* use of crisis houses, if available;
* the client going to stay with supportive friends or relatives who know the issues and can help if the situation worsens;

- people causing stress to the client going elsewhere for a time;
- the use of day hospitals and day centre provision for care and support;
- safety planning strategies such as the handing over of excess potentially toxic medication or potential weapons;
- friends or family staying with the client or agreeing to visit or telephone regularly;
- daily medication administration, support and monitoring by a home treatment team or increased support (e.g. coordinated by a care coordinator including outpatient follow-up and possibly day care);
- coping skills being taught by visiting practitioners;
- any of the list for lower-risk assessments would be equally relevant here.

To make a plan work where there is a risk of harm, everyone involved needs to sign up to it, especially the client. It is not always the case that a client is going to prefer home treatment to admission. The risk of harm can increase if a client perceives home treatment to be a lack of treatment and the resulting feeling of rejection can act as a trigger to harm.

Where admission may be indicated

Admission to an inpatient service may be necessary for some clients for reasons of risk management. This is more likely to be the case if:

- there is little in the way of family or informal carers to support the client;
- the level of intent to cause harm to self or others is high;
- the intent may be variable but there is a plan made by the client where risk is to somebody other than the client;
- carers – whether professional or informal – do not have the ability or desire to manage the behaviour that poses risk;
- if the family or carers have tried and are worn down by their efforts to manage the risk and they need respite (a respite facility would be better than hospital if one acceptable to the client can be found);
- if the client is at risk from others, due to their vulnerability to exploitation when unwell and there is no protection in the home environment;
- if the client is homeless – especially street homeless;
- when whatever could be offered will not significantly reduce the risk of harm occurring and the harm likely to be caused is greater than any harm that would be caused by a hospital admission.

Some patients welcome inpatient admission at certain times because they are accepting of the need for inpatient care and treatment. Others will refuse admission and consideration has to be given to the use of detention under mental health legislation.

There are a few risk management issues to be aware of when such involuntary detention is being considered, whether in or out of hospital. Doctors, key workers and approved social workers involved should carry out assessments under mental health legislation with the benefit of the client in mind. The coordinating practitioner (currently an approved social worker in the UK) has a responsibility to look at possible alternatives to admission and to only use compulsory admission if it is 'necessary and proper in all the circumstances of the case'.[3] Despite this and however humanitarian the professionals feel they are being, detention is likely to feel very different to the client than to them. To face the possibility of having your liberty taken away from you without trial is very threatening. If people feel threatened or scared, the chance of aggressive behaviour and attempts to escape increases, even from people who have never displayed aggression to others before. It is important to acknowledge any distress.

When admitted to hospital, risk issues remain but there are some differences in how they are assessed and managed. These are discussed in Chapter 9.

Case example

Robert, aged 38, lived alone, helped out with a friend who was a builder and had a history of schizophrenia requiring involuntary admission on two previous occasions. His father had had a history of mental health problems requiring detention in secure hospitals but had now died.

He presented late one afternoon at a mental health centre in an agitated and dishevelled state saying that the Japanese army were pursuing him. He was known to staff who took him into a quiet room. Unfortunately, only two members of staff (and a receptionist) were present so the male member went in with him while the other instructed the receptionist to summon assistance – this included the police because of knowledge about Robert's previous history, a psychiatrist and a mental health practitioner (approved to act under mental health legislation). De-escalation by discussion of the concerns he had was attempted and this was done by specific questions about his concerns regarding the Japanese. This quickly extended to discussing a range of paranoid concerns. Robert was quite volatile during this discussion but not threatening to the staff member. An attempt was made to broaden the discussion to include questions about other concerns and home circumstances.

The arrival of the police was managed by the second staff member who quietly explained the situation and entered the room while allowing the door to remain ajar. She was able to communicate that support had arrived and discussion followed of what support Robert might value, ways of ensuring his safety, and, maybe, whether admission to hospital might help. This latter caused Robert to become agitated and the police were asked to assist, and did so. This enabled a mental health assessment to be made safely.

Chapter 5

Emotional difficulties

All crisis presentations will have an emotional component. Emotions are integral to human experience, so whether the person's presenting problem is a thought disorder, eating disorder or other disorder, the fact of being in distress and, in the cases we focus on, in crisis, carries with it a strong set of emotional reactions. These can be of a quite extreme nature and are often commensurate with the client's experiences.

In this chapter we will consider the responses offered to those clients who present with mental health difficulties which are emotional in nature, specifically depressive and anxious presentations. First of all however a discussion about emotional presentations in general is merited given their strong presence throughout mental health crisis work. We wanted to acknowledge different individual, social and cultural attitudes towards emotions, and beliefs about how they should or should not be expressed. Differing beliefs about, and differing levels of being comfortable with, emotional expression can impact on relationships including those between client and mental health practitioner.

Beliefs about emotions

All human beings have emotions as a fact of human existence and they serve various useful, often protective, functions. For example, anxiety alerts the individual to potential threat and mobilises their body and mind to counter it. Depression can be more difficult to understand but may well allow healing and reconsideration, when emotional loss or physical damage has occurred, and may signify to others the need to provide protection against immediate demands. These are normal responses and need not be pathological. Some people may describe themselves as 'emotional', which in common parlance tends to mean they feel emotions keenly and are able to express them freely. Somebody describing themselves as 'unemotional' will still have emotions but they may be more discreetly displayed or given less 'head-space' or credence than analytical thoughts. Some people hold beliefs about emotions and emotional expression being 'weak' or 'wrong' and they may therefore suppress their emotional selves. Keeping strong emotions unexpressed can be an exhausting task causing stress that can lead to a mental health presentation or to physical problems. For example, anger left unexpressed and then internalised can be an issue in depression while stress is cited as a contributing factor in high cholesterol and hypertension, causing heart problems.

There are social and cultural norms that can be very powerful in the expression of emotions. For example, in some cultures a very loud outpouring of grief is the norm whereas in others (e.g. UK middle-class traditions), any loud public emotional expression of grief is more likely to be greeted by others' embarrassment or even disapproval.

Gender plays a powerful role as well. In the authors' (UK white) culture, women are far freer to express emotions of sadness or anxiety than men. This social norm perpetuates the myth that the expression of sadness is not permitted for men. For a man to do something seen as feminine is to invite a challenge to his masculinity. Conversely, it is far more expected that men will express anger than women. A woman who is overtly angry can risk being seen as aggressive by nature – not feminine. There are some signs that these norms are changing, for the better, as they benefit nobody and oppress everybody. In secondary education attention is now more likely to be paid to 'emotional literacy' as part of the curriculum, teaching young people to acknowledge their emotional selves and look after themselves when under stress.

With this in mind, when people present in distress, the presentation of their emotions may not be as it seems superficially. Somebody in tears could be very angry while an angry person could be expressing terrible sadness or fear in the only way acceptable for him or her.

Challenging beliefs about emotions

If a client in crisis holds a strong belief about emotions that is unhelpful to them, it is worth inviting them to identify the origins of their assumptions and to challenge them. This may be something very straightforward. A sensitive response to 'I was always taught it is wrong to cry in public, I am so sorry' might be, 'Look, I see people every day who experience distress and feel no shame at crying about it. The reason we have tissues on hand is because we expect people to be tearful, given what they are going through.'

In some cases, people may have more deeply-held and unhelpful beliefs[1] including, 'being emotional means being out of control', 'emotions are stupid' or that emotions can be right or wrong depending on what others think of them. It can be helpful to convey that, 'Actually, emotions just are as they are and they are OK. Feeling angry does not make you a bad or aggressive person, it is a normal feeling. How you *act* on emotions is important, but *feeling* them is natural and part of being human.'

People needing to do work on managing or coping with their emotions can be referred post-crisis for emotional coping skills work or anger management, but in a crisis the most important point is to validate what the person is feeling, to reflect back their feelings deserve respect whatever they are and that feelings alone cannot hurt anybody else. Where people have levels of emotional distress they feel unable to cope with there is a role in crisis work for looking at a 'first aid' list of what a person can do to cope (see p. 111).

Feeling comfortable about feelings

We said that people vary in the extent to which they are comfortable with the expression of emotions and this goes for mental health practitioners as well as the rest of the population. Some emotions cause particular discomfort for certain people. One person may find expressions of anger very stressful and misinterpret them as aggression. Clients have been heard to say they have been labelled 'verbally aggressive' when they needed to sound off about an issue or an injustice they felt strongly about. A practitioner may feel fine coping with anger but find sadness hard to bear. There is a temptation if someone is expressing seemingly unbearable pain to try to rescue them, to make it stop, even suppress it. This could be by a referral on for counselling or by offering more medication, rather than discussion there and then. That client may want that further intervention but they might also just need somebody to listen and validate what they feel. Whatever the emotion, acknowledging it is respectful to the client.

Practitioners can get to know which emotions they find harder to deal with than others. Self-awareness with regard to this has been established as a part of good therapeutic practice for many years (although perhaps neglected somewhat as health services have become more narrowly task- and outcome-orientated). If we know what we have to work on within ourselves, we are less likely to cause harm to clients by inappropriate or rejecting responses. It is also the case that we as practitioners can be left feeling sad, angry, frustrated, guilty and any number of other emotions and we need to be able to recognise and express these so we do not become subject to stress and burnout.

Emotions and mental health difficulties

There are a wide range of emotions, but we will look in particular at anxiety and depression. Other emotions commonly connected with mental health distress include:

- anger;
- shame;
- guilt;
- perplexity;
- elation.

Anger may present as a reaction to loss or threat in a very similar way to depression or anxiety and much of the discussion following about reactions to these emotions applies. It can present alongside aggressive behaviour (see Chapter 6) but it is very important to note that anger does not automatically lead to aggression and can be closely related to depression and be a presenting feature of mania.

Shame and guilt usually present as components of depression, although they can relate to all mental health problems, and so are dealt with below. Perplexity is present frequently with psychosis and confusional states and so management of the underlying thoughts is generally the way forward (see Chapter 7), although the emotion itself can need a direct response – acknowledging and respecting the uncertainty, anxiety, often fear, associated with it, while beginning work on clarifying the reasons for and nature of the perplexity. Elation is usually a thoroughly enjoyable state which cannot go on too long. However, seeking it by artificial chemical means, through illegal drugs, can lead to crisis presentation (see Chapter 6). Elation can also be a presenting feature of mania but is usually also associated with disinhibition and overactivity, which leads to crisis presentation.

Anxiety, worry and panic

Clients with anxiety often present in crisis because of the intensity of symptoms and fear associated with them. Although a panic attack rarely lasts more than a few minutes, usually insufficient time in which to present to crisis services, recurrent attacks and fears about the causes of them can mean that urgent assistance is nevertheless sought in the aftermath. The support and intervention of friends and relatives alleviates distress in many such situations. But where this is not sufficient, crisis presentation will often then be to primary care services – nurses, family doctors or accident and emergency departments.

It is only when such interventions are not effective that referral to mental health services occurs for advice and anxiety management work. Services vary in whether they are organised to offer this as resource restrictions mean that they prioritise 'severe mental illness'. Anxiety-related crises are not always taken as priority referrals by mental health services whose resources are stretched by work with clients who may be experiencing psychosis or suicidal thoughts. Panic and anxiety can be referred back to primary care or to an outpatient clinic, and time is spent in arguments between the GPs and services about how serious the perceived crisis is. Most anxiety-related presentations can be managed by advice from primary care teams but there are times when the level of panic and anxiety can put unrealistic strain on families and severely affect a person's functioning.

Paradoxically, restricting access can mean that crisis presentations with anxiety symptoms become increasingly common but present later to services.

So they end up having to provide assistance anyway but when symptoms are more deeply rooted, have done more damage and are more severe. Anxiety also accompanies most other mental health problems to a lesser or greater degree so may require crisis management as part of a broader picture.

In screening for the level of need, even where there is no formal depression and no overt physical risks, consideration needs to be given to the social costs of the anxiety. A partner may be unable to go to work or even get a child to school because the client feels unable to be alone. A client may be so agoraphobic they cannot get food into the house or they may be repeatedly ringing for an ambulance, for example, because of fear that they are having a heart attack.

Recent evidence suggests that anxiety and depression form part of the same syndrome such that presentations may vary from time to time, with depressive symptoms prominent on one occasion and anxiety symptoms on another, which has implications for management in the short- and long-term.

How do clients present?

Some examples of its presentation are where:

- A client suffers from persistent headache that leads to attendance, often repeat attendance, at accident and emergency departments, with the fear that they have a brain tumour. Referrals in these cases may come from other health professionals unable to continue providing services that are inappropriate anyway.
- A carer has reached the stage of being unable to cope with a client's anxiety. If anxiety is restricting the client's social functioning, carers can end up being asked to do more and more for the client who may believe they are unable to go out or that they cannot be left alone. Sometimes this can continue for years but a crisis ensues when a carer falls ill or collapses under the strain, or needs to leave the client for other reasons. Referrals may come from child care or education services if carers are young and taking time off school for caring responsibilities or if an agoraphobic client feels unable to get younger children into school.
- Anxiety may coexist with symptoms of depression. Living with chronic anxiety can cause the depression and a suicidal crisis may stem from difficulties managing anxiety. A person may attempt suicide if they are feeling unable to cope with panic attacks, chronic anxiety or with a worry about a particular life problem that has blown out of proportion. In this case the risk assessment is done for any incident or risk of harm to self but the plan then needs to focus on the anxiety.
- There are times when people are referred as having a crisis with

symptoms of anxiety but on assessment they experience a general difficulty in coping with life stresses.

- Clients may present because they have developed coping methods for dealing with anxiety which are now seriously interfering with their functioning (e.g. obsessional ruminations such as counting steps around the house, to counter distress, or avoiding situations which are associated with distress). Usually clients with such problems do not present in crisis but more routinely to services, however such symptoms can lead to partners, families or others reaching 'the end of their tether' and precipitating a crisis by leaving or becoming angry and presenting the client to services.
- A man presents in an agitated state with tremor and sweating prominent. He describes feeling fearful and anxious and unable to sleep. This has been going on intermittently for a number of months. As the assessment proceeds, it emerges that he has been drinking alcohol at levels above those recommended for many years but recently has been drinking less. Other symptoms of alcohol withdrawal then emerge on further assessment.
- A woman presents in a dishevelled condition but expressing very little. She does not appear distressed or anxious but vacant in expression, seemingly in a dissociative state, and very slow and distant in responding to questions. Answers are vague while sometimes looking flustered. It gradually emerges that she had a past history of significant trauma. Memories of this have just been reactivated by hearing that the perpetrator has returned to live locally.

Box 5.1 lists common symptoms of anxiety.

What can you do?

When anxiety rises to the point where urgent intervention is needed, it is particularly helpful, if possible, to work with the client's family, friends or carer as well as with the client. This is so that when the client is left alone, the most helpful approaches can be reinforced by people around the client. Carers are usually grateful for advice on what to say or not to say to somebody. They can also provide valuable information during the assessment (see Chapter 2) about current circumstances and past coping abilities.

To work with a client presenting with anxiety or having a panic attack, begin by establishing what the anxiety is about, as part of the assessment. If the client is too agitated to provide much information or complete the assessment:

- ask about what are they frightened of;
- establish whether their fear is proportionate to the situation;
- if it is not, discuss this with them, letting them tell you why they are so

Box 5.1 Anxiety symptoms

- *Physical*:
  - muscles tense;
  - startle response;
  - tiredness and weakness;
  - aches and pains; headache or backache, or pains in the arms or legs or chest, or in any other part of the body;
  - stiffness;
  - appetite reduced (or alternatively, increase in 'comfort eating');
  - stomach tightens up, abdominal discomfort and 'butterflies in the stomach';
  - diarrhoea;
  - increased desire to urinate;
  - hair 'stands on end' and causes 'goose pimples';
  - heart rate increases, blood pressure rises;
  - palpitations – awareness of heart beat;
  - breathing rate increase ('over breathing');
  - tingling in the fingers and toes;
  - uncomfortable awareness, even tightness, around the chest;
  - dilated pupils, blurring of vision;
- *Psychological*:
  - feeling anxious;
  - fear of physical harm, going 'mad', fear of failure or fear of damage to status or a relationship;
  - fear of the unknown;
  - apprehension and uncertainty;
  - feeling of being under excessive pressure;
  - irritability;
  - loss of libido;
  - loss of interest in activities and hobbies;
  - loss of ability to selectively concentrate;
  - loss of memory or dissociation;
  - worry and rumination (obsessional thinking and rituals);
  - sleep disturbance;
  - depression.

fearful and eliciting from them reasons why they need not be as immediately fearful; *guided discovery* of their concerns and weighing up the reasons for and against them can reduce anxiety, allowing a full assessment to occur and can be therapeutic in its own right;

- if this isn't working, go directly to use of a relaxation technique or (sometimes better) distraction by asking about relevant but non-stressful issues, to take the client's mind off their current symptoms.

It is important to *explain* anxiety. Even if a client has had information about the way anxiety works and how it physically affects the body, it is worth offering to go over it again. This is particularly the case if the person is having recurrent panic attacks and is seeking a lot of help from general medical services, despite investigations having demonstrated no identified cause for physical concern. Written material to take away on the subject is also useful (see Appendix 2).

It is also useful to teach some basic anxiety management techniques. Simple breathing methods can be taught quickly and can help a person who is feeling out of control. An example of this is 'square breathing' (See Box 5.2).

Box 5.2 Square breathing

The client is invited to look at a square (e.g. at a window). Starting at the bottom left-hand corner they breathe in to the count of five until they are looking at the top left corner. They hold their breath to the count of five across the top, moving their eyes down to the bottom right. The breath is then let out to the count of five. The person counts across the bottom of the square for a count of five before breathing in slowly at the left hand corner again (see Figure 5.1).

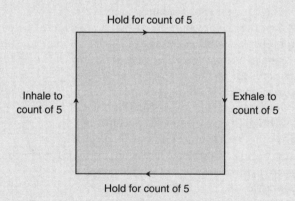

Figure 5.1

Doing this with a visual focus aids concentration and slowing the breathing rate down should relax the body and prevent hyperventilation.

Any breathing exercise will do if it slows and regulates the breathing. The client may know one they have used to cope in the past but have got out of the habit of using. It may be necessary to use techniques like this to bring the client down from high anxiety to a state where they can work on formulating a plan with the mental health worker.

Some patients, especially those who are worried already about their breathing (e.g. that it may stop) find breathing exercises are not successful as they increase the focus on breathing and sometimes exacerbate panic. So modifications of progressive muscular relaxation techniques can help. This involves working around the muscular groups in the body, tensing and then relaxing them. Simply guiding the person through this process can break a vicious cycle of panic and anxiety – if they are able to cooperate. Where they have difficulties or when they are in a public setting, sometimes just concentrating on one muscle group can be successful.

It is now time to review and begin to tackle life stresses. Problem-solving and cognitive behavioural approaches are equally valid with anxiety presentations, once the immediate distress is reduced. Obvious routes for help, support and reassurance are partners, friends and families and, perhaps, doctors or counsellors, and these alone may be sufficient to alleviate the anxiety. If there is a particular reason for the anxiety, it may be possible to do something about it and discussion is probably the best way to decide what is wrong and how it can be changed. The client may feel that the problem is insoluble or a situation unchangeable but there may be some way around it which they have not thought of. It may even involve admitting something to themselves, such as their marriage being over, which they have been trying to deny because it is discomforting and may have implications for changes in the future. Change in itself may increase anxiety and the client may stay in the same tense and worrying situation rather than go through the trauma of changing it for something different – however necessary that change may be.

Similar issues to those occurring in depression can occur with anxiety. The relevance of vulnerability, particularly personality issues such as dependency, guilt, obsessionality and asociality, may need to be explored and disentangled in this context. The negative thoughts involved may differ at this moment (e.g. focusing on feelings of being threatened, either individually or in relation to physical or mental health), but the methods to deal with them are those described with depression.

Work with carers is often crucial as their anxieties can reinforce those of the client. The parents' attitudes to the client's problems should also be considered as their anxieties can be very important as maintaining and even precipitating factors. Illness or death of parents or someone close to the client can precipitate fears of a similar event in the client. Parents' fears of illness in the client can equally increase *their* anxiety. Similarly, conflict with carer or parent can be a factor in raising anxieties but may not be identified through assessment unless it is thorough and includes a good assessment of relationships. Advice about family or partnership counselling may be appropriate – crises for all parties can sometimes lead to such options being explored where previously avoided. Unassertiveness can present as anxiety or depression and need direct intervention – identifying the issue and a way forward can assist in crisis resolution.

Use of alcohol or drugs can complicate the picture. Withdrawal symptoms commonly present as anxiety but the steps described above are unlikely to be of much immediate benefit unless the withdrawal is completed and sustained.

Dissociative states appear to be a reaction to overwhelming distress and anxiety. They may be associated with depersonalisation and confusion (see Chapter 7) and may have a defensive function – rather like shock – reducing the intensity of the emotional experience. Gentle calm questioning and discussion can gradually reveal the problems and assist in working with them, as described previously.

Self-help options for anxiety

There are many self-help options available for people suffering from anxiety and introducing them to these possibilities can be a valuable outcome of a crisis presentation. Most adult education departments run classes for either relaxation or managing stress and anxiety. There are a number of self-help books available on the topic[2] and a various national associations concerned with different phobias or anxiety in general. One example of a particularly useful organisation is No Panic (www.nopanic.org.uk). No Panic has a help-line and sufferers can join for a small fee and gain access to leaflets, videos, telephone recovery groups and information over the internet. Triumph Over Phobia (www.triumphoverphobia.com) is another organisation that has support groups in a number of locations across the UK. The anxiety management techniques described above can help, as can physical activity, from a walk in the park to to serious exercise in a gym. Exercise uses up excess adrenaline and relaxes the body.

Identifying individual ways of relaxing is most effective and sometimes this involves rediscovering those used in the past. Even after talking and thinking it through, the client may remain or become again quite tense and anxious and, in that situation, it is important to find ways of relaxing. It may be that listening to a record, chatting with friends or playing a sport or game will help. However, through lack of practice, the ability to relax may become 'rusty' and learning a relaxation exercise may be useful. Alternative forms of relaxation and exercise including yoga, reflexology, aromatherapy, t'ai chi and acupuncture can have a calming effect on anxiety. Such complementary therapies are now available in most areas but are usually only available privately at varying cost.

Avoidance

Anxiety is reinforced by avoiding the situation, thoughts or individuals that are the apparent source of the fear. Avoidance damages confidence and stops the concerns being dealt with. While times of crisis may not seem to be the appropriate moment to try to deal with long-term patterns of avoidance, if we are to make the most out of crises – using them to facilitate change – they can be the time to begin the process of dealing with issues left undone. A rationale for attempting to deal with anxieties rather than flee from them needs to be developed. It is also necessary to work with the client on changing negativity and hopelessness. The feared situation may seem overwhelming – too frightening. As the relationship develops, it becomes possible to discuss what they fear might happen and debate the likelihood, severity and possible consequences of this happening. With further time and continued relation-ship development, discussion may allow 'the worst thing that could happen' to be discussed in the same way and 'decatastrophised'. Exploration of the formerly unknown and unnamed usually clarifies and reassures.

Using medication

Medication has a limited part to play in managing mental health crises involving anxiety and panic. More sedative anti-depressants may help in the medium and longer term, with sedation and sleep improvement often coming quite quickly, so they may be worth adding to psychosocial measures. Benzodiazepines do little more than postpone and exacerbate crises although they may be useful as hypnotics for a brief period to re-establish a better sleep pattern. However, their longer-term dependency effects and general thera-peutic ineffectiveness can lead to agitation, especially where supplies are threatened, and seriously impair self-belief and confidence. Longer-term benzodiazepines are sometimes considered, such as Clonazepam, but their value is debatable. Anti-psychotics are also sometimes used but again evi-dence for them is not strong. Crisis periods again may not seem the time to begin discussion of withdrawal from benzodiazepines but by identifying one exacerbating problem and providing a plan for supported – and relatively painless – withdrawal, clients may see hope for a future without dependence on medication and with less of the negative effects entailed.

Case example

Nathan, aged 33, had presented to the accident and emergency department five times in the last two weeks with chest pain. Each time he was sent home following examination and investigation but he continued to be distressed and in pain. He was seen by the duty mental health practitioner after his family doctor insisted. His initial presentation was reluctant. He was annoyed that he was being ignored and was saying that he was 'not crazy'. The assessment unearthed a variety of symptoms as well as the chest pain including breathless-ness, tingling and diarrhoea. 'Well wouldn't you be anxious if you were getting pain like I am and nobody is doing anything about it,' was Nathan's response.

As he gradually told the practitioner about his circumstances and personal history, it emerged that Nathan had been under a lot of work pressure to complete a major project and had been working very long hours. It also turned out that his father had died quite young of a heart attack and his mother was also very concerned that Nathan might be at risk himself. Nathan was not sure what was wrong with him but found the pain he was getting difficult to understand and tolerate. As he told his story, he became more relaxed and noticed that his symptoms were easing. He was given a full description of the effects of anxiety on the body and agreed that whatever else might be happening, he was certainly anxious.

There was not much he could do immediately about the work pressures. He wanted to finish off the project which he was due to complete within the next couple of weeks. But he agreed that he would moderate his work demands, if necessary by speaking to his boss. He was not keen to have medication but agreed to see his family doctor for a sedative anti-depressant if the situation did not improve. He took information about anxiety away with him and would come back in a week or two to discuss progress. He also

---

Box 5.3 Anxiety checklist

- Do a full assessment including personal and family history.
- Explore current pressures.
- Get a full description of symptoms; when and how they started.
- Don't start talking about anxiety until assessment and formulation is completed.
- Discuss and name the specific fears the client has.
- Draw from the client what they understand by anxiety and supple-ment it as needed (possibly with written material).
- Discuss their views about whether anxiety is involved and if so how.
- Work out a plan to deal with any sources of stress.
- Find out how they like to relax and encourage them to do so or to try alternative methods.
- Consider use of complementary therapies.
- Describe and give brief training in a simple relaxation technique.
- Consider if medication is likely to be useful and arrange for the client to obtain it if so.
- Provide contact point and review date.

thought it would be useful to convey what they had discussed to his mother and, if she wasn't reassured by it, to bring her along next time to discuss it further.

Depression

Most people will experience symptoms of what mental health services call depression at some point in their lives. They go through a period of feeling low with loss of energy and concentration, lack of hope for the future, sleep disturbance, appetite changes, irritability and overwhelming feelings of misery and tearfulness. For most this is an unpleasant experience which they work though with the support of relatives and friends. For some however it becomes overwhelming and they present in crisis.

Depression is not a term used in a very precise way. Most clients who present in crisis say that they feel depressed because this is their way of generally describing negative feelings associated with adverse life events and distress. Some may be more discerning about differentiating between feelings and will describe stress or anxiety as the prominent problems. Others may deny being depressed at all because they associate it negatively with failure or inadequacy, or being ungrateful to others, or even for religious or cultural reasons. Their presentation may then be of physical symptoms or deterioration in performance or behaviour with denial that anything is wrong with their mental health. Differentiating whether the person is depressed, anxious, confused or angry, or any combination of these emotions, can be helpful in deciding which of these feelings to work with, or in which order and how to do so.

There is an increasing awareness of depression generally. Family doctors are prescribing more antidepressants than ever before and counselling services are becoming increasingly available. This means that initial treatment for depression will often have commenced prior to the crisis presentation and this will influence assessment and management.

What is depression?

When a client presents in a crisis with a depressive disorder, their features are likely to be perceived as severe (see Box 5.4). The severity of the depression is likely to involve negative self-punishing thoughts, perhaps thoughts provoking feelings of intolerable guilt or worthlessness such that the person may not feel able to live with them. Or else their lack of energy may have dragged the person down to a state where they can barely move or function: so-called psycho-motor retardation. There may be an overlay of anxiety with the person suffering chronic agitation. There can also be psychotic symptoms when people are low, such as visual or auditory hallucinations or delusional beliefs, especially paranoia, inadequacy and guilt.

Box 5.4 Depression

Symptoms can vary considerably but may include:

- *Feelings*:
    - depressed, anxious, angry, confused.
- *Behaviour*:
    - isolating, neglectful of self and others, erratic, slowed up, impulsive, argumentative, hostile, drug and alcohol misuse.
- *Thoughts*:
    - content: negative, guilty, non-coping, hopeless, suicidal, paranoid;
    - processes: worrying, confused, forgetful, poor concentration, obsessional, hallucinations.
- *Physical symptoms*:
    - sleep problems: not getting off, waking in the night and early morning;
    - appetite: reduced or increased;
    - fatigue, lack of energy.

Presentations vary and a list of symptoms can be very broad and helpful only in determining that the person is depressed and to some extent the degree of depression. Classification systems tend to be unhelpful. They consist of a dimensional description – mild, moderate, severe – with or without psychotic symptoms. In practice, describing depression as mild to a client is unlikely to enhance engagement as depression by its nature, certainly when presenting in crisis, rarely feels to the individual as 'mild'. Psychotic symptoms are also not 'all or nothing'. When do thoughts of guilt move from being reasonable to being unfair to being delusional? Voices experienced are often initially recognised as illusions and accompanied by insight into their association with the person's mental health problems even when quite loud and insistent. And where does PTSD, usually involving severe depressive symptoms, fit? Terms like agitated depression or even melancholia are descriptive in terms of severity and type of symptoms but mean little in terms of treatment and prognosis for the future.

It may be more helpful to think of how and in whom depression presents and assess and manage accordingly. It is now clear that adverse social circumstances can lead to depression whether related to a specific experience, as in PTSD, or more chronic problems (e.g. unemployment or relationship breakdown). The response to these depressive symptoms depends on the person's individual strengths and vulnerabilities: severe stress, combinations of stressors or lack of social support can overwhelm a person and produce a range of severity of symptoms. Where somebody previously has had difficulty coping with life stressors, the severity of the stress and effect of withdrawal of social support may have an effect at a much lower level than for someone who has developed self-confidence and resilience – although the crisis presentation may look the same. Similarly, for example, someone who is quite perfectionistic and finds disruption to their life difficult to handle, may also present in response to lower levels of stress and may be more likely to develop significant associated guilt.

Presentations of depression can be very variable but it may be useful to consider three particularly common patterns as they can help guide management:

- 'social depression': response to social triggers including the effects of other physical and mental health problems in someone who normally copes effectively;
- 'dependent depression': response is modified by previous difficulties coping (e.g. excessive dependency on others or difficulties in forming supportive relationships);
- 'guilty depression': response is modified by excessive need to control their environment, expressed as perfectionism.

The predisposing vulnerability factors (see Chapter 3) can significantly shape presentation as can those stressors which precipitate the crisis. Assessment therefore needs to account for these areas. How the person coped before the crisis is as important as the factors directly involved now.

Crisis presentations in depression often hinge around the risk of suicide and this always needs to be assessed (see Chapter 4). Thoughts of suicide are very common with depression. As symptoms become worse, clients may consider acting on their suicidal thoughts if they come to believe that they have no reason to stay alive. Depressed clients can come to believe that others may be better off without them as the negative thoughts that characterise depression take a stronger grip. Mental health professionals may become involved following a failed attempt at suicide as the person recovers in the local general ward. Or they may be involved when the person telephones for help, feeling that they cannot go on, or if friends and carers report signs that the person may have suicidal intent.

Another presentation with depression that can cause alarm and distress is self-harm. This may or may not be allied to suicidal thoughts and it is best not to assume that one flows from the other (see Chapter 6). Some people self-harm in a way which endangers their life and a self-harm incident may be the initial 'go' at attempting suicide. A client's intent when they harm themselves is a crucial indicator of the response required. Some clients may harm themselves by cutting, without any aim to end life. Some talk of needing physical pain to distract them from the intolerable emotional pain they feel. Others use self-harm in an effort to reduce tension or agitation.

Staying with the concerns about the risk to life and emotional well-being that depression can cause, self-neglect can also be severe when caused by depression. This is particularly the case when the client concerned has withdrawn to the extent where they are refusing food and especially fluids. Human beings can keep going for some time without food depending on age and state of physical health generally. When clients stop drinking anything there is more immediate concern as this can compromise kidney function. Signs of dehydration include dry mouth and flaccid skin, and confusion. The assessment and management of the above concerns were discussed more fully in Chapter 4.

There are other negative outcomes that can be produced by untreated depression that are more gradual and less visible until they emerge as crisis. As somebody becomes more depressed they are likely to withdraw socially and may feel unable to carry out the most basic of tasks. There are large variations in how people react to depression. Some people may be able to function at a very high level for periods while experiencing massive problems with sleep, suicidal thoughts and tearfulness. Sometimes the mere belief that they have no choice propels people out of bed to feed their children and get them off to school or to, somehow, get to the post office to pay bills. Other people may find these tasks become beyond them as their depression increases in severity. People can neglect to claim benefits, fail to renew sick notes for their employer or put off paying rent or bills. People who have a strong and close social network may be more protected from the negative effects of this loss of social functioning. People who live without other supportive adults may get into all sorts of problems, with the risks of losing income, getting into debt or even potential homelessness if rent is not paid. These practical difficulties then serve to feed the depression as the threatening letters come piling in, reinforcing the person's belief in their own worthlessness and inability to cope. The presenting crisis may therefore be a practical problem which needs sorting out as an initial intervention.

Depression and children

Sometimes the crisis for the depressed client may be related to their children, either as reported by them or as a referral to mental health services from children and family social work teams. People with symptoms of depression who have children can feel less and less able to provide them with the care they need. Many people cite their commitment to their children as being what keeps them going and individuals can be inspirational in the way they manage to parent in spite of severe mental illness. However, for some people, at times when the depression may be very physically restraining, it can be hard to do the multiplicity of tasks involved with parenting. Professionals need to be sensitive to children's needs when assessing a depressed mum or dad even if the referral has not come from a child care source, especially if the family has no support or relatives nearby. A depressed parent may feel unable to mention concerns about poor school attendance or neglect for fear of being punished rather than supported. Older children may be taking on more of the care of younger children if a parent is unwell and a referral to young carers' services could be a relief to the depressed parent as well as to the young carer (see also Chapters 2 and 4).

Changes in levels of support

Crises may occur when others' circumstances change. A bereavement or separation may present as an event which in itself is distressing and assessing and managing the grief involved will be the primary focus. However, where crisis involving such loss events presents to mental health services, a key issue is often the loss of support that is entailed. That person might have been the client's sole or most important confidant or have provided valuable practical support. Alternatively, and this may complicate the assessment, the relationship may have been difficult, fraught and critical and resulted in anxieties and subsequent mixed emotions when the loss occurred – which in turn may cause confusion, guilt and distress.

Understanding crises

The causes of depression are important for crisis assessment because knowing what triggered an episode can give clues as to appropriate management. Developing a formulation (see Chapter 3) can help in this. Drawing out the vulnerabilities, strengths, triggers and maintaining factors can begin to clarify the development of the crisis. Beginning to understand the relevant thoughts, feelings, behaviour and physical symptoms within this environment can take assessment forward into intervention and a crisis plan (see Figure 5.2).

So, the initial stressor may be environmental, for example a client may have persistently noisy neighbours who play music through the night and whose kids are bullying the client's children. Maybe the client has recently lost by death or divorce a more assertive partner who used to deal with these problems. The client may get little or no sleep and be chronically tired and tense (physical reaction) leading to doing less in the day and keeping the children indoors (behaviour). This can lead to self-critical thoughts such as 'I can't cope' or 'I am failing my kids by not sorting this', in turn leading to feelings of anger, sadness and despair. The negative thoughts and feelings keep the client awake thereby increasing the tiredness and everything escalates. The five aspects are interlinked and are important to hold in mind because when intervening in a crisis the focus of the intervention can be on one or more of the five areas in order to break the cycle of depression. The crisis may arise

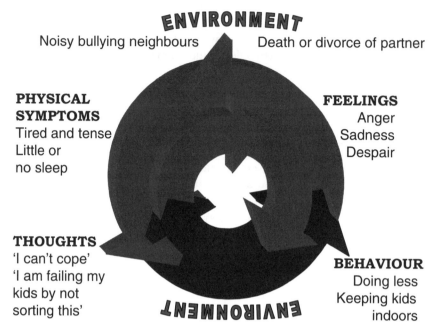

ENVIRONMENT

Noisy bullying neighbours   Death or divorce of partner

**PHYSICAL
SYMPTOMS**
Tired and tense
Little or
no sleep

FEELINGS
Anger
Sadness
Despair

THOUGHTS
'I can't cope'
'I am failing my
kids by not
sorting this'

ENVIRONMENT

BEHAVIOUR
Doing less
Keeping kids
indoors

Figure 5.2 Inter-relationships in depression

when the client presents at the family doctor's surgery feeling unable to carry on and convinced their life is no longer worth living.

What can you do?

A good assessment can be therapeutic for the client in that they will have been able to tell their story and that alone can be cathartic. Understanding how their depression began can reassure the client that their symptoms are not a reaction of which to be ashamed or that need be overwhelming. Assessment as a process should also be helpful in engaging with the client.

Safety considerations

Given the correlation between depression and the possible negative outcomes outlined above, the initial work after the assessment (and usually done as part of it) has to be concerned with the immediate safety and well-being of the client and those around them. Once the client and as appropriate their carers have explained the situation, the initial questions to consider are:

- Is there any evidence the client is likely to commit suicide in the near future?

- Is the person neglecting themselves to the point where their physical health could be damaged?
- Are the client's depressive symptoms preventing them from carrying out caring responsibilities (e.g. towards children or older relatives) that they formerly undertook and do alternative arrangements need to be made for those needing care?
- Are there any other immediate risks to themselves or anyone else?

If the answer is yes to any of these questions then a risk management plan needs to be agreed by all involved. This would include the client and carers having contact numbers should the situation deteriorate.

Finally, are any urgent practical arrangements necessary (e.g. a phone call to a housing office or a benefits agency) to ensure the client has a roof, food and essential utilities? Support may need to be arranged for children or relatives from family or friends or from social services, or from a combination of these. A few telephone calls may need to be made to reduce external stressors (e.g. lack of cooking facilities or heating, provision of food or broken doors or windows repaired). There is really little point in attempting an intervention to manage a crisis until the person you are working with has the basics: physical safety, food, housing and warmth.

Problem-solving approaches

The next step in intervening with a person in distress is to plan a strategy to deal with the presenting problem or problems (see Box 5.5[3]). It may be that the person has come for help at this particular point because they can no longer cope with feelings that they have had for a very long time. Alternatively there may have been a recent and sudden stressor. The initial approach is about looking at solving immediate problems, developing ways of managing those that are impending and finding coping strategies for the future.

Helping the person resolve their problems involves initially being clear together about what the issue is or issues are. What is reasonable and achievable

---

Box 5.5 Problem-solving stages

- Clarification and definition of problems.
- Choice of achievable goals.
- Generation of solutions.
- Choice of preferred solutions.
- Implementation of preferred solutions.
- Evaluation of whether actions are effective.

to overcome or solve the problem? What is the best way of doing this? A very basic start is by identifying resources to assist the client and writing a list of their supports and stresses. These lists can be as varied as you like. An example might be:

My supports

1   C. (wife): listens, is supportive, holds tablets.
2   Sam and Leroy, mates: I cannot tell them how bad it is but can use them for company on a good day, watch TV etc.
3   Fishing: gets me out of house.
4   Car magazines.
5   Bed, hiding under duvet.
6   Talking to my sister on the phone.

My stresses

1   The kids: if they are being hectic.
2   Dad: goes on all the time when I see him.
3   Thoughts of going back to work.
4   Debt.
5   Garden: needs doing.

If someone can identify what helps them or has helped them in the past and what makes them worse, they can be encouraged to make use of their supports and to avoid or else plan to resolve their stresses. It makes sense in a time of heightened distress to avoid seeing people who upset you and to increase the time spent with people who are supportive. If someone is identified as having a carer role as part of this process (in our example the client's wife) then there is an opportunity here to involve her in the process so she knows what will help. It is also an opportunity to put her in touch with carers' services, supports and helplines.

Environmental issues

Some of the stresses in people's lives are going to be precipitating factors in their depression and could exacerbate or at least maintain the distress if left unattended. The use of problem lists can be helpful in managing mental health emergencies in order to establish and prioritise what requires immediate intervention. Even when clients present saying their only issue is that of wanting to commit suicide, there are often massive social stresses going on for them that led to these feelings. Some can be resolved and some cannot. Some will need immediate input and some will wait.

Stresses arise in all areas of life, for example:

- *relationships*: with partner, children, parents, friends or neighbours;
- *workplace*: overwork, bullying, unemployment, fear of job loss;
- *financial*: debt, benefits problems, bills disputes;
- *housing*: homelessness, disrepair, eviction, noisy or unfriendly neighbourhood, isolation;
- *legal*: court appearance, being a witness or a victim of crime, seeking asylum or immigration;
- *social*: being a victim of racism or homophobia, being harassed, isolated or unsupported in life;
- *health*: being in chronic pain, loss of previous abilities through poor health, diagnosis of a physical illness, harassment or exclusion through being a mental health client.

There may be numerous issues but what the client identifies as being the most prominent are the ones to initially work on. Having identified resources and ways of proceeding, the next step is to act on them or to set a rough timescale for completing them in. Sometimes immediate action is possible and necessary. Support could be accessed to help a client with financial advice, or to seek help following discriminatory harassment from neighbours, or to look for housing for a homeless client. People will vary in their ability to cope with and resolve issues depending on the level of their depression and previous coping abilities. Other problems cannot be so easily sorted (e.g. a long-term relationship problem between the client and their parents). Such problems are better acknowledged and then a way of managing them worked out. In a mental health emergency, helpful discussion in this instance might be to do with the amount and type of contact that is necessary between the client and their parents and whether this can be reduced or at least changed, for example, when, where or with whom they meet, while the client gets over the current high level of distress. More thorough work connected with this relationship would be more appropriate for longer-term post-crisis input. Often having an achievable plan can reassure the client and lead to resolution of the crisis. Completing the plan may take time but identifying a way out and beginning to feel hopeful can have a rapid effect on depressive feelings.

As the process of dealing with the problems proceeds, evaluating the effectiveness of each action can, where successful, assist in building confidence and self-esteem. Where actions are not, or only partially, successful, it may be possible to learn from the experience and try other ways to deal with the situation.

Where problem-solving isn't working

Often the obvious direct approach to solving problems doesn't work or the client is reluctant to take it. It may be that:

- all the problems have not been identified or managed effectively – reassessing and reviewing with the client the initial conclusions and crisis plan may lead to fresh approaches;
- the nature of the stressful events is such that beliefs about themselves are affected (e.g. they are wrongly blamed by other family members for their mother's death);
- the symptoms of depression directly interfere (e.g. paranoia leads to isolation and increased fears);
- earlier factors in the client's life have affected their ability or style of coping with stressful events and circumstances (see 'dependent' and 'guilty' depression, p. 11).

Earlier we looked at how the environment interacts with people's thoughts, feelings, behaviours and physical reactions and this provides a route to disentangle and work with these more difficult situations. An explanation of the interactions (drawn from cognitive behaviour therapy) can be of benefit to the client and use can be made of these different aspects of life to add strategies to somebody's plan to understand, deal with and protect themselves from depression.

Behaviour and goal-setting

Behavioural activation, i.e. increase in activity, has been shown to be a particularly effective component of cognitive behaviour therapy in depression and so it is reasonable to focus initial attention on this, although not in isolation from the influence of thoughts and feelings. A depressed client is likely to have a reduced level of activity, for example, causing them to feel unable to contact friends or family or do activities they previously found enjoyable. It also becomes harder to do what is needed to manage the environment (e.g. to tell children to clear up, to go to work, to do shopping or housework, to report much-needed repairs to the housing office or to tell neighbours their behaviour is causing stress). This in turn affects mood as the inability to act leads to amplified feelings of sadness, guilt and thoughts of failure.

Setting goals so that clients get a feeling of achievement can in turn help mood. A very depressed client needs to set goals that reflect what he or she is able to do. Goals set that a client cannot achieve do more harm than good. It is therefore generally better to ask the client themselves to suggest goals rather than set them yourself. So for one person, their goal might just be to get out of bed and get dressed each day. A client with more energy may set a goal to walk to the local shop. Clients may also have goals that work on alleviating some of their life stresses, possibly with support from a friend or a professional (e.g. visiting a benefit office to sort out financial issues).

The nature of depression is that it often varies in intensity during the day with most people finding mornings more difficult. It is reasonable to build this consideration into setting goals and also to consider together whether there are ways of improving, for example, mornings. Avoiding decisions of any sort at that time can be helpful so that a routine is set and an attempt made not to question it as doubtful ruminating simply aggravates depression and inactivity further. If any decisions need to be made for the next day, making them the evening before can help. Discussing plans with a carer or mental health worker can also help in weighing up the reasons for and against even apparently simple and straightforward decisions.

Depressed clients who manage to do activities that they formerly found to be fun can be quite despondent if they now find that they derive no pleasure from them. They may take reassurance from being told that this is one of the cruelties of depression, but that by doing them, they can get a sense of achievement and so may feel better than they would have done if they had stayed in bed and done nothing. Initially *it is mastering the activity rather than getting pleasure from it that is the goal*. Sometimes it is worthwhile asking the client to rate and write a timetable of favoured activities. This can be valuable in demonstrating to someone in crisis that ways forward with their problems are possible. Subsequent referral for more formal cognitive behaviour therapy can follow.

Working with negative thoughts

Some people manage their lives effectively despite feeling depressed and they can keep doing what they need to do. However, they can still be plagued by negative thoughts about themselves that perpetuate low mood. People describe their experience of depression as akin to being inside a glass box – they appear to be functioning from the outside but are unable to communicate their negative thoughts and feelings. Where previous experiences are relevant, 'I can't cope' or 'I'm a failure in life' may be beliefs which are key to making progress. Identifying them as issues can focus attention on crucial areas and lead to meaningful strategies which in turn instil hope for the future.

In a crisis there are some tactics that can be brought into play. Let the client know that negative thoughts are symptoms of depression and are common to many people. Leaflets about depression and lists of common thoughts[4] can reinforce this. This approach can begin to challenge the 'objective truth' of the thoughts in the client's eyes and work against feelings of guilt and isolation.

Invite the clients to challenge negative thoughts that they have about themselves. If they are invited to provide proof for the 'fact' that they are stupid as well as proof for the 'fact' that they are not stupid, they can arrive at a less punishing view of themselves. As a note of caution, clients in crisis may need help to do this as it can be hard to find proof that counters negativity when they are riddled with self-loathing. Looking at issues such as 'I'll never cope' or 'I'll never succeed' and breaking down what these mean can often be done even in apparent crises. Make it specific: 'What is it you need to cope with?' 'What are you trying to succeed at?' 'Let's just try and deal with your immediate situation – there'll be time to look at longer-term problems later' and 'How can we deal with this specific problem?' It may be necessary or helpful to write a positive and negative balance sheet about 'what you have coped with and not with' or 'successes and failures' with prompting and then debate or problem-solve relevant items. Often depressed clients magnify negative aspects and minimise positive ones, get them out of context, take things too personally or overgeneralise – identifying this when it occurs can begin to lift mood and build hope for the future.

Ask the person to write down ten good things about themselves. They are likely to find this nigh on impossible, particularly as we live in a culture where self-praise is frowned upon as 'boasting'. Useful prompts to this are to keep it simple, take nothing for granted and write what friends and family would say, as we are generally kinder to others than we are to ourselves.

Writing down one positive thing every day is good for self-esteem. Again this can be simple (e.g. 'I cleared up today even though I didn't feel like it'). Homework that encourages self-praise can work against all negatives.

Mood

Any or all of the above can be put into a plan for a client and will often begin to lift their desperation somewhat and resolve the crisis situation. The client can be invited to rate their mood out of ten on a regular basis to see how their actions affect how they feel. However, rating mood is not appropriate in all cases – for example if motivation is very low – and can be insensitive and confirm 'uselessness' in some cases.

Some clients may present with their strong emotions paradoxically being the seeming or a contributory cause of their distress. They need time and validation to begin to recover and simply listening for a relatively short period may be important. A basic brief exploration of why they are feeling the way they do can enable the issues involved to be mapped out and also lead to some relief.

There are also some clients for whom emotions are overwhelming and even this basic problem identification proves too difficult. In these circumstances, after an initial period of expressing their feelings, some way of helping them move toward resolution is important. Simply continuing to be tearful, angry and distressed – with or without expressions of self-harm or suicide – in itself becomes increasingly distressing and feels more and more hopeless.

Where this crisis is part of a pattern of repeat problems in coping with overwhelming emotions, the client may benefit from knowing that ongoing work to help them manage their emotions can be very effective, instilling hope, especially when their problems are putting them at risk or sabotaging their ability to manage their lives. If a client has already done such work in the past then this can be drawn upon. The client may have a list of what or who can help them which they have with them or is in a crisis plan on file. They may have done more formal emotional coping skills work (see Chapter 6) involving skills of radical acceptance, mindfulness, self-soothing and interpersonal effectiveness. If they have, then they can be encouraged to identify what has worked for them and to continue to practise these skills, however they are feeling, so they are better prepared for the next crisis. More usually in a crisis, the client will have done none of these things and although there may well be grounds for referral for this sort of work post-crisis, there needs to be a way of helping the client immediately.

Many clients experiencing these difficulties receive a label of 'personality disorder' (see Chapter 6) but may also have symptoms of depression, as listed above. For that reason, many of the coping strategies discussed elsewhere are relevant. The client is likely to need a plan that is geared to helping them manage when their emotions feel out of control. A basic formulation that acknowledges past difficulties and trauma is validating and supports the client to put current feelings into a context. A list of potential triggers can be useful, though for some people it may be as much their own anxiety and interpretations of outside events that trigger powerful distress. What all clients in this situation can use is some work to draw up a coping strategy: a list of what to do the next time, or sometimes in the current situation, when they begin to feel overwhelmed. Such approaches include:

- *Relaxation techniques.* It only takes a few minutes to teach and practise one with a client.
- *A list of 'treats' for the person.* Such as a favourite food or a hot bath or aromatherapy oils, anything that leads the person to value themselves.
- *Friends or family to ring and talk to.* Such people need advice as to what to say. Sometimes, if they are (understandably) worried, their anxiety can rub off on the client who may lose confidence in his or her ability to cope. As always, working with the carers is essential here.
- *Ringing a helpline.* Such as the Samaritans or an out of hours service if one exists.
- *Having something else to focus on.* Such as doing a basic task. If the person is calm enough to be introduced to the art of 'staying in the moment', or mindfulness, then some initial practise at this could be beneficial. An exercise can involve 'making a cup of tea'[5] in which the person focuses their attention on each step in the process – going to the kettle, hearing the water go in and feeling the weight increase, putting it on, going to the cupboard, choosing a cup or mug, and so on. They should be encouraged to practise this regularly with different tasks, which it may be helpful to list, when not in distress so it becomes useful when needed.

- *Knowing that others can feel as they do*. Knowing about national helplines (e.g. SANE, Samaritans, Depressives Anonymous) and the existence of therapy for people with these sorts of issues can inspire hope, even if the waiting list for therapy is likely to be long. If the client has suffered past traumas such as sexual abuse or violence, they can also be given contact and helpline numbers where they can get help.
- *Sensitive use of humour*. This can affect mood directly and have an energising effect, especially where mood is not too low. If you know your client well enough to sense when it might be appropriate, the use of humour can induce a sense of pleasure in some circumstances. The act of smiling lifts mood. Some people, as part of their crisis or prevention plan, use videos of favourite comedians or particular films that will make them laugh. It is about forgetting problems and negative thoughts for a period at least.

Physical aspects

Physical symptoms can present and cause anxiety to clients with depression and need to be identified and managed (see Chapter 8). The thoughts that clients get can be negative or fearful and these need to be explored and worked with. Tiredness and low energy interact with mood and behavioural issues. Physical illness, especially pain, can also be a potent source of depression, acting as an aggravating or precipitating stressor. Applying a problem solving approach to it will often include the family doctor or liaison with other physicians involved or needing to be involved in the client's care. When depression is particularly severe, beliefs about change in body functions, shape, even the existence of organs (Cotard's syndrome) can occur.

Some clients can improve their energy levels and mood via physical exercise, which also encourages healthier eating patterns. While going to the gym may be far beyond a depressed person in crisis, a walk around the block or a swim may be enough to relieve tension, improve sleep and be beneficial to mood. Of course a depressed person who is used to vigorous exercise when well could be in a position to make themselves do this however low they get.

There has been work done on the relationship between 'food and mood' and some clients may be interested in this though it does not seem to have reached mainstream services or been proved to have a major impact on outcomes. Poor diet and unappetising food certainly does not help. It makes sense that good eating will help physical symptoms of depression and clients interested could be directed to relevant literature.[6]

Sexual function is often affected by depression and medication can be used to treat it. Clients may fear that such changes in function will be enduring and will need to be informed that this is not the case (unless there are other contributory reasons than depression and anti-depressants), but that sexual function is often one of the last symptoms to remit as depression lifts.

Effects on memory can also cause concern. Concentration is reduced in depression – often because thoughts are elsewhere, worrying about specific issues or simply the fact that the person feels low. This affects memory for events and is further affected by general negativity. Clients may fear that they are dementing (depressive pseudodementia) or have some other damaging process occurring in the brain. Again information about the effects of depression can help to allay such concerns.

Some clients are reluctant to take anti-depressant medication, however severe the presenting symptoms. This may be influenced by past and recent press coverage of the side-effects of psychiatric drugs. Others may already take an anti-depressant. For clients not taking anti-depressants, there are usually advantages in doing so where significant depressive symptoms present, as is usually the case with crisis. Explanation that treating the physical symptoms of depression can improve sleep and give a person the energy to eat or bath, or even socialise, can be crucial in assisting the client to achieve other goals. It can also have a beneficial effect on negative thoughts which can be amplified by managing stresses and by cognitive behavioural work directly focused on them.

Depression and alcohol

People experiencing the very distressing symptoms of depression may try to alleviate those symptoms with the use of illegal drugs, or more commonly with alcohol. There is a strong cultural pull in the UK towards solving your problems with 'a pint of beer' or usually rather more. Specific drinking customs vary internationally but alcohol taken to dull feelings of depression and anxiety is almost universal. Use of alcohol in particular can increase the symptoms of depression that people use it to relieve. They can then get stuck in a vicious circle of alcohol use and depression that can spiral downwards.

When people present to services in crisis with symptoms of depression they are likely to be asked about their level of alcohol intake. Excess usage may be diagnosed prematurely as a primary alcohol problem and they may then be referred on to substance misuse services for help. The situation may then arise where people find themselves being 'batted' between two services as the substance misuse team sends the client back for help with the depression. Working collaboratively can reduce the likelihood of this happening and agreed, perhaps joint assessments, can establish the most appropriate way of working with a group of people in whom risk of suicide is elevated. In many cases, it becomes impossible and pointless to try to identify which came first, the depression or the alcohol use, as both will need addressing.

Clients with depression often speak of feeling that mental health professionals can be blaming and unsympathetic if they admit to drinking alcohol. There have also been cases when issues which are clearly not related to alcohol are minimised as stressors causing depression as professionals see the alcohol but not beyond. Of course, the life stresses that contribute to depression can also drive somebody to drink. The two are intermingled and a judgemental attitude is unhelpful and prevents engagement in working with either issue.

Dealing with alcohol and depression

Where alcohol is an issue, clients first of all need straightforward non-judgemental information about alcohol or other substances that they use. Alcohol is very likely to increase the severity and symptoms of a depressive illness. It can also reduce the effectiveness of anti-depressant medication. The use of alcohol also increases the risk of self-harm. People feel less inhibited when drinking so are more likely to attempt and commit suicide. Clients need support to be able to act on this information. If somebody has used alcohol as their main support for a long time, it is going to be difficult to alter that pattern of behaviour. They may need access to a range of services or helplines.

Sometimes clients say they are left with the impression that the *only* problem is the alcohol. If clients stop drinking alcohol, it will help their recovery from depression but the symptoms of depression remain to be treated and identifying what caused the depression in the first place is still vital. When clients stop drinking there is no perceived buffer against life and its social stresses. Stopping drinking does *not* equate with recovery and it is demotivating to service users to suggest that it does. It is merely that once a client stops drinking, recovery has a chance to begin.

Using medication

If the client presents with moderate or severe symptoms of depression and is not being treated with an anti-depressant, one generally needs to be prescribed. As such medication has not been shown to reduce depressive symptoms for two weeks or more, it will not have an immediate effect on the symptoms although it may well have an effect on anxiety and sleep disturbance at an early stage. It is also likely to have effects by beginning to instil hope in the client and their carers that something can be done to improve their symptoms and this can have a major impact in relieving crisis. If symptoms are less severe, the evidence is more limited as to whether anti-depressants are beneficial and their use needs to be weighed against other considerations. The selective serotonin reuptake inhibitors (SSRIs – e.g. Fluoxetine, Sertraline, Paroxetine and Citalopram) are generally used as first-line medication and seem to be relatively free of side-effects, with complaints of nausea and stomach upsets occasionally occurring. However, there is some emerging concern that agitation, hostility and suicidality may be adverse factors and warning about these effects is necessary. There does not appear to be any difference in effectiveness between the individual SSRIs but some possible difference in sedative properties (Fluoxetine and Citalopram seem to cause this least). Interactions with other drugs being taken also need to be considered. St John's Wort is also used in mild to moderate depression and may be more acceptable to clients, but interactions are again important to beware of.

The widespread availability of anti-depressants generally means that most clients presenting with depression will already have been prescribed one at an earlier stage in the development of their problems. Should you change or supplement it? There is no research evidence that changing to another drug within the same or another group (except possibly to serotonin and nor-adrenaline reuptake inhibitors (SNRIs)) leads to improvement although it is very common practice. A case can be made for it if additional effects such as sedation or reduced side-effects is the aim. There is limited evidence that changing to an SNRI, Venlafaxine, may have added benefit and this can be considered although it needs to be under specialist supervision and contra-indications and precautions considered. Change to a tricyclic anti-depressant is also often considered, usually to one with lower levels of toxicity in overdose, such as Lofepramine. Again some evidence exists that Amitryp-tiline or Imipramine may be more effective but the potential adverse effects, especially in overdose, are such that caution is needed in their use. Supple-mentation by mood-stabilising drugs is also frequently practised (e.g. use of Lithium, Thyroxin or Lamotrigine), and by anti-psychotics or benzo-diazepines. The latter is certainly problematic, although Clonazepam, a longer-acting drug, may be useful where agitation is associated and can act quite rapidly. Addition of an anti-psychotic, especially those which also reduce agitation such as Olanzepine or Quetiapine, may also be an option. Any such addition of medication in crisis requires review once the situation has stabilised – it is very easy for medication to increase step-by-step, crisis by crisis.

Before increasing or supplementing medication, it may be worth consider-ing the potential effect of psychosocial interventions. This can often mean that such changes are unnecessary or at least minimised as a plan for dealing with current stressors and negative thoughts is set out. Potentially, changing medication can take the focus away from situational changes which may be necessary but uncomfortable. Medication change may seem an illusory quick fix which simply postpones action – or it may aid action by improving mood and motivation.

Case example

Surrinder, age 58, was divorced five years ago but has remained the main carer for two children aged 24 and 18. Both have left home, the youngest very recently. Surrinder has worked for many years as a general nurse. She is now under pressure from her older siblings to take over the care of their disabled father. Surrinder was physically abused by their dad when she was young.

She has been off work with symptoms of depression and presents in crisis, tormented by feelings of guilt that lead to her believe she should take her own life. Her plan was to attach a hosepipe to the car exhaust. Her protective factor restraining her from proceeding was the effect on her children.

Intervention

- Naming the problem was the hardest part for Surrinder who was used to giving support, not taking it. She was encouraged to identify and name the distressing thoughts she had – about being a failure because of her divorce, being a bad person for not taking her dad in and being useless as she felt unable to work. Gentle exploration of the issues allowed mental health staff to help Surrinder reapportion blame for the situation away from herself and accept her feelings as understandable.
- Gathering support was difficult for Surrinder as she was reluctant to share. However, she confided some of her distress to a nursing friend and colleague and was pleasantly surprised by her offer of company and a listening ear. Surrinder wrote to her family explaining she was unable to help with her father at the moment due to her own health problems, which avoided the issue, but bought Surrinder some time to work out how she really felt about it and what she wanted to do.
- Surrinder was not well enough to work but was encouraged to engage in other activities she had previously enjoyed, including seeing her children.
- She was sleeping poorly, lying awake plagued by guilt. She was already taking an anti-depressant but was given a more sedative one to reduce her agitation and aid her sleep. She was encouraged to do more during the day to make her physically more tired.
- As she had expressed a plan and lived alone, Surrinder was seen as a high suicide risk and was monitored daily for a period by a home treatment service. They let her talk and were alert to thoughts that might indicate that she felt her family would be better off without her. After a discussion on safety planning, Surrinder and a support worker moved the hosepipe to the loft so it was not readily access-ible if she had a bad night and was impulsive. She had a phone number to ring 24 hours a day in case of worsening thoughts and heightened distress.

Box 5.6 Depression checklist

- Fully identify:

    o   symptoms of depression;
    o   risks;
    o   stressors;
    o   what might help.

- Develop formulation and crisis plan:

    o   respond to risk;
    o   problem-solve stressors – especially immediate practical measures;
    o   brief focused work with negative thoughts such as guilt (see Appendix 2)
    o   develop a relevant and realistic activity schedule;
    o   identify social supports and how to access them;
    o   revew use of medication.

- Provide contact point and review date.

A client's perspective

The chapter explored a wide variety of issues, offering good guidance for practitioners. The models of practical help could easily be applied to a variety of support workers and indeed would be employed by myself as a debt counsellor. I feel however that there was brevity in the detail of support available for isolated clients.

Dee

Chapter 6

Behavioural problems

Problems or concerns about behaviour are frequent presenting issues in crisis. Assessment should determine underlying causes, such as depression or psychosis, but misdiagnosis is very common and can be dangerous in terms of not intervening where risk to self or others is present, or at least mean that effective treatment is not offered at an early stage. It is also possible for inappropriate intervention to exacerbate behavioural problems.

Behavioural presentations include:

- self-harm or neglect;
- aggression;
- overactivity;
- disinhibition;
- agitation;
- rituals;
- wandering;
- substance misuse;
- compulsive behaviour (e.g. gambling);
- demanding behaviour.

Presentations can be symptomatic of virtually any mental disorder: mania or hypomania, depression, panic or psychosis, and also of physical illnesses, 'personality disorders' and 'out of character' behaviour in someone without so-called personality issues, especially under the influence of drugs or alcohol.

It is very easy to become judgemental in relation to assessment and management of behavioural presentations and this can distort assessment – jumping to conclusions is common where behaviour appears to be 'deliberate' and therefore it is assumed that the person is not entitled to health and social care. It can be difficult to determine whether somebody is fully responsible for their actions, or that their actions are influenced by illness or by their early life experiences, and it can be very easy to get it wrong. The response offered in each of these situations differs, but deciding that one or other is more morally justifiable should *not* be the function of services and their representatives.

The most important issue to assess is whether the behaviour presenting is part of a mental health or physical problem or a longer-standing behavioural problem linked to emotional distress and relationship difficulties, often labelled 'personality disorders', or is nothing to do with any of these. A good assessment of personal history as well as history of current and past illness and contact with mental health services is most useful in determining this. Assessment of childhood and early adulthood with a focus on the relationships formed or absence thereof and then subsequently in later life, can provide the basis for understanding the individual's capacity to form relationships and the issues involved with them. Where such relationships, in work or home, have formed and been sustained, behavioural symptoms presenting are quite likely to form part of a current mental health problem. Where this hasn't been the case:

- if onset of problems was in adolescence, there may not have been time for such relationships to form and a mental health problem such as schizophrenia may be presenting – which can also be associated with shyness and isolation in childhood;
- personality problems make people more vulnerable to mental health problems so both may be present;
- personality issues may be the key element in diagnosis but a crisis has arisen leading to the current presentation.

It is important at this point to stop and discuss the term 'personality disorders' as this is quite often the diagnosis that has been given to people who present with behavioural symptoms in crisis. It is a term that we feel uncomfortable with for two reasons:

- The concept of personality comes very close in common parlance to describing the core of a person's identity. Being told that your personality is somehow disordered feels like criticism and condemnation of the individual in a judgemental manner.
- The term is frequently taken to imply that, if it is the person's personality which is disordered, then it is not a medical matter and a client's problems are, by definition, not amenable to treatment. This model of mental health means that many distressed individuals can be excluded from services or made to feel that they have no right to a service. In fact, it is likely that medical interventions are of limited use, although medication can help clients to manage depression and other distressing symptoms. However, psychological and social interventions can be helpful to clients, improving their abilities to cope with and understand their distress, and

there is evidence that people can experience less distress (or 'get better') with such input (see below).

Clients will present in crisis with an assortment of possible personality disorder diagnoses in their notes and we need to take these into account, acknowledge them and describe how these types of problem could impact on a client's behavioural presentations. On many occasions they will not be aware of the diagnosis or be aware but disagree with it.

It may be more helpful to think in terms of difficulties with relationships rather than personality disorder in this context:

- People who have few relationships and don't seek them (known in diagnostic terms as 'schizoid') may be more vulnerable to behaving 'oddly' and concern can be expressed about them in terms of perceived risk to others or of neglect to themselves.
- People with relationships which tend to disrupt easily but who may be striving to make new ones (known as 'borderline') can present as very distressed and sometimes impulsive.
- People who come to depend excessively on relationships with others can't cope when needs are not met or when the person depended on cannot meet those needs, leaves or dies. Such clients express this as being depressed, anxious or simply by demanding emotional or other support ('dependent').
- People who tend to be rigid or fixed in their ways can have their relationships disrupted by this inflexibility ('obsessional'). The consequence of change in their lives, including failures in relationships, is for them to present as depressed and sometimes anxious.
- People who may form relationships but move from one to another with a seeming disregard for the effects of their behaviour on other people are known as 'antisocial'. Eventually the consequences of their actions may catch up with them and they present as depressed, anxious, substance misusing and can be impulsively suicidal or aggressive to others. They may also be looking for support in avoiding facing consequences (e.g. criminal charges).

Many clients who receive a diagnosis of borderline, antisocial or dependent personality disorder in particular are in fact suffering the consequences of trauma, especially childhood sexual abuse and emotional or physical neglect. Their disrupted relationships and extreme level of emotional distress are understandable when seen in the light of what they have been taught to believe about themselves – for example, that they are powerless, that they are responsible for their own abuse, that they are therefore guilty, shameful and not worthy of help. Indeed it has been formulated that for those who suffer trauma and abuse the responses practitioners call 'maladaptive' are in fact 'logical, rational and necessary' responses to their abusive experiences.[1] The beliefs and emotional distress that abusers cause put the abused person at risk of mental health problems of many kinds, but this is often not enquired about or acknowledged by a medically-focused approach. Holding some appreciation of the reasons why clients may appear self-punishing, rejecting of help or distorting of boundaries can make practitioners more understanding. Clients may believe they should be punished, that all helping relationships are unsafe, or have had their relationship boundaries so distorted as children that they have never learnt what constitutes socially acceptable boundaries in relationships.

Given the social stigma attached to mental health issues it seems cruel to be saddling clients who have suffered abuse with an over-generalised label of being 'personality disordered' when what they are experiencing is often a reaction to chronic trauma. However, many such clients are in the mental health 'system' and present asking for help in quite desperate need and/or are referred to services because the behaviour they use to cope causes anxiety and distress to those around them. The behaviour of some clients can also make them vulnerable, putting them at risk, either of physical harm to themselves (even death), or of losing relationships or ending up in the criminal justice system, depending on their behaviour. People have a right to help in these situations and it is to mental health services that many turn in crisis. We therefore have to live with the risk of clients feeling that their experiences are being pathologised but try and work with this risk in mind and, most importantly, ensure that mental health services do not 'replicate the abuse' in terms of attitudes and interventions.[2]

Some behavioural presentations can represent mental health problems even where they appear to be deliberate and irresponsible (e.g. gambling, alcohol misuse or increased sexual activity with a large number of new partners, which is very out of character). Such behaviours can be symptomatic of depression or mania. They can also be an acceptable lifestyle choice. The behaviour in its own right therefore needs to be seen in the context of a comprehensive assessment. Where this behaviour is new and out of character, it may form part of a mental health problem. Self-harm and aggressive, eccentric, impulsive behaviour can all manifest themselves in this way. If a diagnosis of a mental health problem is made, treatment of that disorder may be sufficient to alleviate the behaviours but they may also need action in their own right.

Self-harming behaviour

Any act of self-harm needs to be considered in terms of risk of further and more serious suicidal acts (see Chapter 4). Having made that assessment and instituted appropriate immediate management, while continuing to keep it updated, deciding what is responsible for the self-harm determines treatment.

If it was due to depression alone or as part of another mental disorder, management of that disorder is appropriate. The immediate consequences of the self-harm also need to be managed. Repeated lacerating can be difficult to deal with, although newer surgical glues have made this easier to physically handle. A sympathetic, non-judgemental approach from staff is crucial.

The evidence that people who self-harm repeatedly can be helped is growing, with use of longer-term interventions like dialectical and other cognitive behaviour therapies and also psychodynamic approaches based on interventions in day hospitals.[3] Some clients also find support through self-help groups or by getting therapeutic help to work on past abuse issues that may be precipitating the self-harm. This is very important in terms of prevention but may seem of little value in the immediate crisis.

Engagement may be difficult – the client may expect a negative reaction for the reasons considered above about past experiences and take retaliatory action before it arises, for example, by expressing anger, dismissiveness or increasing attempts to self-harm. The situation may already be getting out of hand with the client's anger and agitation being transmitted to others. This is especially the case where those around the client are unused to such circumstances or have learnt seriously maladaptive ways to respond. The approach made is therefore crucial – first impressions matter. Gender is also important. Often an approach from a woman to a female or male user will be less threatening but not necessarily so. Individual reaction matters – and often you have little choice about who is available to see the client.

Being strenuously non-judgemental is very important – and difficult to fake. Convincing yourself that an empathic approach to someone who appears to be self-destructing is appropriate rather than using a more 'behavioural' stance is not always easy. It may help to consider what it is like to feel distress and rejection which seems intolerable – and to have the means to get rid of it or at least reduce it quickly. This is what taking an overdose of sedative medication, consuming excessive amounts of alcohol or causing lacerations does. Even more extreme behaviours like fire-setting can have a similar anxiolytic effect. The short-term effect of these behaviours can be profound but, of course, can also be hazardous. It can be helpful to share your understanding of why the person self-harms with them: 'I understand that self-harm reduces some people's distress at least at the time – is that what is happening to you?' You can acknowledge the distress, understand the reason for the methods being used but *then* begin to explore alternative ways of handling that distress.

Discussing precipitating factors can help alleviate distress. Some of these may be recent (e.g. an argument with family members, investigations or a court case involving abuse) and sometimes past experiences of significance emerge during the assessment process. These can seem so overwhelming, unpleasant and even horrific that you may fear that discussion of them might seriously increase distress and consequent risk. However, avoidance of discussion can lead to even greater desperation and increased self-harming behaviour. The safest course is usually to be guided explicitly by the patient: 'What you are talking about sounds very distressing – if you want to talk with me now about it, that's fine. But if not, or if you don't want to continue, please say so.' If they show any hesitancy: 'On the other hand, I don't want you to feel you have to discuss it in detail now – we can talk about it later or I can arrange for somebody else to talk with you.'

If the circumstances are such that sufficient time cannot be made available, saying this and ensuring that such time can be found as soon as possible can prevent deterioration. Being stopped from talking about these key issues can be felt to be rejecting and devaluing and so increase distress and self-harming behaviour.

The worst case scenario is that the questions are not asked or statements not believed so that the client and assessing professional get an inaccurate formulation of the origins of the problem and the client has their feelings of self-blame for the current situation reinforced. A client may not choose to share information about any past abusive experience, and this is their choice. However, the fact that a mental health practitioner has asked the question gives the client permission to raise it at a later time if they so wish.

Tactics for dealing with distress include specific behavioural techniques, mindfulness and also constructive and cooperative engagement. Behavioural techniques may involve distraction or assertiveness (even rehearsed within the crisis interview – e.g. specific comments or responses to husband, family members or work colleagues). An introduction to mindfulness techniques may be helpful. This means encouraging the person to essentially be in, and aware of, the moment: 'participating with attention'[4] to the task in hand and not applying any judgement to thoughts and feelings, just acknowledging that they are *there*. The acceptance of distressing feelings can be discussed, and an emphasis on tolerating distress and not judging it can reduce the level of distress over time and so reduce severe self-injury. Remaining in the moment can be helpful when clients feel their emotions are out of control; focusing on the concrete world around them stops the mind 'running away' and it puts the client back in control. Mindfulness skills are not easy to master but there are exercises that clients can be given to assist them.[5] In crisis situations this is particularly relevant if the client has had experience of using these skills in therapy and needs a reminder to make use of them now, and it can also instil hope by demonstrating to them that there are ways of helping them that can be developed for the future.

Engagement in dialogue about key problems and developing a realistic plan of action can also be very effective. Agreeing that their life at the moment is 'shit' but being able to discuss ways of making it less so can engender hope for the future, counteracting the overwhelming negativity. Fear may be an important component and being able to allay this can help (e.g. the client may fear that a past assailant is going to attack them or that they are going to be put in prison or hospital). Where such fears are warranted, straight discussion and analysis of the reasons for the fear can allow negotiation to occur and safety measures or alternatives to be devised.

Another option is to work with the client to produce a checklist of what may ease the need for the behaviour. This can then be kept by the client, if they wish, for future crises. A list may include such things as names of people to phone, a safe place to hit out and express anger without injury, ways to relax or alternatives to cutting such as snapping an elastic band against the wrist or crushing ice. It may also contain a list of what to avoid doing. 'Do not drink alcohol' may sound like obvious advice but given how culturally acceptable it is as a relaxant it is worth suggesting that clients consider abstaining when in distress. This can be explained as being because in their circumstances, alcohol is likely to increase distress and risk. It is wise not to assume that they have heard it before as it may not have been fully explained in a non-judgemental way – they will tell you if they already have such information and do not want it again.

If someone is self-harming or threatening to do so, attempting to physically intervene is almost always counterproductive and can be dangerous – trying to remove a razor blade or knife or even a bottle of pills can easily escalate to more extreme uncontrolled behaviour. Waiting and discussing may take time but will almost always be successful. If intervention is deemed necessary for the safety of others or because behaviour is becoming increasingly risky to self, it needs to be well prepared and discussed by the team involved to have a chance of success.

Case example

Gemma presented when she was 25 to accident and emergency having seriously lacerated both her wrists. She was distressed and angry. After initial attention had been given to the wounds, she told the staff that she was leaving and did not want to see anyone from mental health services as she had had bad experiences with them previously. At that moment, the mental health worker – Laura – who had already been asked to see her, walked into the cubicle where she was. Laura immediately introduced herself, commenting on the fact that she was from the local mental health team and had heard that Gemma wasn't impressed with the contacts with services she had had previously. She expressed concern at how distressed Gemma seemed and how significant the damage to her arms appeared, offering to do what she could to help – if there was anything that Gemma thought would be appropriate. Assessing the risks involved was not easy alongside trying to develop a non-confrontational relationship. She managed to engage Gemma in a discussion of her current home situation – where she was living and how satisfactory it was – and what sort of supports she had. It turned out that she did have parents close by, but relationships were distant, and one good friend.

With continuing discussion, Gemma's distress seemed to reduce and she provided sufficient information for Laura to decide that there was no immediate risk of suicide. The self-harm had been in the context of extreme frustration and anger and had occurred previously in similar situations. Although she did not provide details, it did seem likely, from her reaction when asked, that there had been events in her early life which were continuing to trouble her. Eventually it was agreed that Gemma would call her friend, go home, but meet for a fuller discussion with Laura at a time agreed in a couple of days time. Laura described briefly some of the things that might be offered – a chance to talk things through and maybe look at some alternatives to self-harm.

When do you increase support up to the level of admission to hospital? Admission is not helpful in most circumstances where self-harm has been repeatedly occurring, although risk assessment should always be made. Occasionally, early on in the development of a relationship with the person, it may be necessary to admit particularly if there is no home treatment option available or risk is uncertain. Where someone has repeatedly self-harmed, direct statements, such as a threat to commit suicide, are not usually followed through but it can be difficult to feel comfortable with leaving someone or telling someone to go who has the means and apparent drive to do so. Self-harm can also be dangerous and careless of life such that someone may not mean to seriously harm themselves but do so 'accidentally'.

In the longer term, a consistent approach can be very effective, although this is not always immediately accepted by the client. For example, they may be asking for hospital admission in crisis, but in the longer term this reinforces non-coping and ultimately lowers self-esteem. In addition, the circumstances of acute inpatient wards can lead to the exploitation of vulnerable individuals. Therefore, in some cases it may be more appropriate to seek alternatives such as intensive home treatment or respite care.

When a relationship has developed and full assessment has been made over time, management of repeated self-harm can evolve to the point that when the client presents in crisis, plans are available to help them and perhaps avoid the need for admission. Admission can become addictive because responsibilities are removed and nurses can provide a very supportive and nurturing environment. However, dependence on admission reduces self-esteem and coping skills so unless risk is high it is best avoided. Increased support can be an alternative, for example, from a home treatment team or via extra visits from a support worker or care coordinator. Having a contact point and/or telephone number available can reduce crises and ideally the contact should be someone known to the individual rather than an emergency duty system. Even an agreement with the assessor, care coordinator, psychiatrist or therapist to ring the client back as soon as possible after they make contact can help. Often the person tests this out by ringing to see if a response is forthcoming, and if one is they tend to use the facility very infrequently.

Establishing a crisis plan and looking towards longer-term support and intervention can begin with resolution of the immediate crisis. Where the client is repeatedly presenting in crisis, it is very important to put in place follow-up measures such as regular visits/appointments and reviews, to bring stability to the situation and prevent the client and services from going round in frustrating and counter-productive circles.

Use of medication

Medication can be of some value although there is a very limited evidence base for its use and there are dangers in providing harmful substances that can be taken in excess. Medication is however prescribed remarkably often with many clients taking substantial amounts, and often many different types of drugs simultaneously. Negotiation about what would be helpful can be therapeutic even if it is eventually decided that medication would not be very helpful and isn't prescribed. Anti-depressants may be of limited, but not immediate, effect, but simply the offer of *something* to help can instil hope and be useful. More sedative anti-depressant medication (e.g. Mirtazepine or Trazadone) can be useful in reducing the anxiety and agitation patients experience and should improve sleep. There is some limited evidence for SSRIs being effective but they, and tricyclics, may cause a paradoxical increase in suicidal behaviour. Anti-psychotics may help with agitation and also any psychotic (or psychotic-like) symptoms, such as voices, visions or extreme flashbacks. Mood stabilisers are often used, however they seem only to be effective in reducing aggression without much effect on mood, they have dangers in overdose and are contra-indicated where pregnancy is a possibility. Benzodiazepines are more problematic: short-acting drugs can disinhibit and cause greater distress, although occasionally they may help in extreme situations. Where used as hypnotics, they may have a place for re-establishing or at least improving sleep patterns. Medium- and longer-term benzodiazepines are only useful if used as part of an alcohol or drug detoxification regime.

Case example

Jenny, aged 23, had suffered from diabetes for a number of years and had a history of repeated self-harm involving overdoses and saying she would inject herself with excessive insulin. This had led to repeated admissions to psychiatric units and general hospitals. Despite the apparent danger, she did not in fact significantly endanger herself, although said that she would do so. She had had an unhappy but not abusive childhood but now had no contact with her family. Support from a mental health nurse and psychiatrist was provided and validation of her obvious distress at the time of self-harming given. She agreed to attend an emotional coping skills group (based on Linehan's dialectical behaviour therapy). She nevertheless continued to present in crisis to the local accident and emergency department and was in danger of losing her accommodation because the staff at the group home felt unable to cope with her behaviour. An agreement was reached between the care workers that admission to hospital was not helpful and was exacerbating the behaviour, but regular and scheduled dedicated time to discuss issues would be helpful. Jenny accepted the reasons behind the decision but nevertheless continued to present.

Admission to the psychiatric unit stopped after discussions by crisis staff with the Jenny about how unhelpful this had been in the past, and after coordination with the inpatient unit. When Jenny said that she would proceed to take an overdose of insulin if discharged, this was discussed in terms of 'we are sorry you feel that distressed but we believe there are alternatives to harming yourself and we don't think that admitting you is the right thing to do'. The quite extensive services available to Jenny were discussed. For a period she was able to secure admission to the general hospital but communication with them eventually led to this being discontinued or, where they felt investigation of whether an overdose had been taken or not warranted admission, this was very brief. Over the next few months, the self-harming behaviour stopped and work on psychological issues and developing relationships, self-esteem and confidence progressed.

Aggressive behaviour

Verbal hostility is quite commonly associated with crisis presentations, physical hostility less so, but it can clearly cause significant problems. Whether expressions of anger are justified needs to be considered before assuming it to be unwarranted verbal hostility or aggression. Physical aggression is probably never justifiable, at least in this context, but may have been provoked by circumstances. Has the person been kept waiting without explanation? Has someone been hostile, rude or patronising to them? Are they very frightened? Has the assessment process raised past issues that have raised strong anger feelings that then get displaced onto staff? Anger is a common presenting problem and can be a component of;

- depression;
- anxiety;
- psychosis;
- mania;
- substance misuse;
- personality disorder;
- 'righteous indignation'.

If a client's anger is justified by the current situation (righteous indignation), it is obviously important to attempt to compensate for this with an appropriate explanation or apology, and if necessary assurance that action is instituted in relation to the perpetrator of the offence or that it is bought to the notice of the appropriate authority.

In each of the other categories above, the stress of a client's situation may have a non-specific aggravating effect but other symptoms of the syndrome can enable a diagnosis to be arrived at through an appropriate assessment.

Certain factors can be particularly important in weighing risk. These overlap significantly with those for self-harm but deserve reiterating.

- *Substance misuse*:
  - the direct influence of alcohol and stimulants leading to disinhibition and sometimes paranoia;
  - cannabis tends to be more sedating or at least reduce drive towards aggression by its direct effects, but if it produces a psychotic state it can cause paranoia and hallucinations;
  - opiates and alcohol also sedate but withdrawal effects can lead to agitation and aggression and a demand for more drugs and the means to obtain them.

- *Personality disorder*:
  - impulsivity and limited appreciation of the effects of behaviour on others can be a serious problem.

- *Psychosis*:
  - paranoia can make people fearful and unpredictable;
  - commanding voices in themselves are probably not associated with serious aggression but can make someone irritable and argumentative; beliefs that they are being made to act on commands and are so doing may occasionally be a more serious risk.

- *Anxiety and depression*:
  - can lead to irritability;
  - can be associated with psychosis (as above).

- *Past behaviour*:
  - if someone has acted aggressively in the past they are that much more likely to behave that way again, or worse; extreme jumps in behaviour (e.g. from shouting to stabbing with a knife) tend not to occur but from threatening with knife to stabbing might.

What can you do?

Safety considerations take precedence and these can be achieved by use of management of aggression techniques which are sensitive and calmly applied. Immediate responses are:

- Ensure safety – in the rare circumstances where someone is actively physically aggressive, restraint may be necessary but should only be attempted by suitably trained personnel. Where such personnel are not immediately available, may be overwhelmed or weapons are being used, the situation will need to be held or watched until appropriate support is available.
- Enquire about the reasons for the anger being expressed; this can be done even when restraint is taking place.
- Examine what can be done about these reasons.
- On the basis of ongoing assessment, determine whether underlying mental or physical health problems exist and can be managed in their own right.
- Seclusion, although this is used rarely, in inpatient settings.

When working with someone presenting with aggressive behaviour, different levels of intervention deserve consideration and may be worth discussing as alternatives to the behaviour being presented:

- Discussion about current personal difficulties, with specific examples from daily life, can be used to engage the client in dialogue and begin to focus them on a problem-solving approach as an alternative to impulsive and counter-productive behaviour.
- Skills-based approaches which involve developing appropriate assertiveness and anxiety or anger management can be used.
- Evidence of effectiveness of treatment of 'antisocial personality disorder' using cognitive behaviour therapy is not good, but it has been more successful in relation to sex offenders in the criminal justice system.
- Work on 'core' changes in personality has been the objective of psychotherapeutic approaches over the years but there is little robust evidence of effectiveness in reducing symptoms or changing behaviour. There may be a danger of distracting the person from the key objective of behaviour change. However, work on specific issues (e.g. repetitive negative problems in relationship development or the enduring effects of child sexual abuse) may be reasonable to discuss.

Expertise in managing and modifying aggressive behaviour has been particularly developed in the probation service and they can be a valuable ally. Community multi-disciplinary groups involving police, social service departments and (where relevant) mental health services can liaise with one another to oversee care of all individuals who may present a risk of violence or sexual offending. For those at most risk, in whom mental disorder is apparent, admission to special units may be necessary.

If you can develop a dialogue where mutual respect can be seen to exist and clear unambiguous honest discussion occur, situations where hostility is developing or has occurred can be defused. Criticism and patronising attitudes and statements tend to make things worse as can increased emotion and certainly any suggestion of threat. Reasoning about the circumstances and possible outcomes – both positive and negative – can be done cautiously and allows confrontation to move towards collaboration.

Use of medication

Medication can be very valuable in managing immediate risk where this may be the result of a mental health problem. Sedation by a short-acting benzodiazepine such as Lorazepam can be rapid, safe and effective in the short term. Interactions with other medication including alcohol need to be considered. Where psychotic symptoms are apparent, Haloperidol is the antipsychotic most usually used, although newer drugs may be given orally. Haloperidol, Lorazepam and, recently, Olanzepine are also available as injectable preparations. Where crises are repeated, use of short-acting depot injection medication such as Zuclopenthixol acetate ('Acuphase') may be appropriate, but only according to strict guidelines. Use of longer-term depot injections would be more appropriate where crises are continuing to occur. Dealing with underlying reasons for aggressive behaviour remains very important as over-reliance on medication can increase frustration and paranoia. It is very important that medication is used as part of a broad approach to management and seen to be as such by clients and staff. Side-effects of medication, especially where used in high doses over longer periods, can seriously aggravate the situation. Akathisia in particular can increase agitation and aggression and dystonic reactions (muscle spasms) can be frightening and cause increasing paranoia.

Case example

Charlie had been admitted to the ward under mental health legislation with a police escort. He had a long history of schizophrenia, drug misuse and anti-social personality disorder. Within hours, he was storming around the ward demanding discharge and threatening staff with violence. Over the next couple of hours, the ward manager spent time intermittently walking around with him discussing his concerns. There were a number of these which were gradually listed as the perceived unfairness of being brought into hospital, his lack of cannabis, his father's abusiveness to him and having no accommodation of his own. Each was taken in turn: his rights to appeal were explained; cannabis could not be supplied, but the sooner the situation calmed the quicker he would have leave and be able to obtain some, if that was what he decided; he need not see his father if he did not want to and ward staff could explain this to his father if he wished; finally they would get some housing department forms to fill out and arrange for him to see the unit's accommodation officer as soon as he got back off leave. This approach, along with regular doses of Lorazepam (for the first couple of days) and Haloperidol led to a degree of stability, albeit with occasional eruptions.

Overactivity

Verbal and physical overactivity – excessive talkativeness and continuous movement – can be due to:

- personality characteristics;
- anxiety (see Chapter 5);
- mania (or its milder form, hypomania).

Distinction is made by determining:

- background, especially from collateral assessment;
- how long activity has been present;
- if it is increasing.

Mania presents with:

- persistent elevated mood – elation; can be mixed with depression, irritability, anxiety or hostility;
- unrealistic or grandiose ideas; paranoia;
- increased interest in socialisation, food and sex with disinhibition;
- distractibility;
- rapid cycling mood and behaviour;
- poor judgement and insight;
- lack of sleep;
- may not eat or do so voraciously.

Although in theory the distinction should be straightforward, it may not be, especially in the early stages of an episode. Often people who experience mania have quite lively, talkative personalities or are prone to anxious garrulousness. It becomes easier to assess extremes when the person becomes psychotic and expresses beliefs which are clearly delusional in terms of their bizarre nature, but early intervention is designed to reduce the chances of the client reaching that level.

What can you do?

Careful assessment can determine whether someone is going 'high' or not and in the early stages this can be detected by the person themselves in many cases. A belief in your own uniqueness and specialness is a positive attribute supporting self-esteem, but a belief that you are extra-special – more so than others – can begin to verge on the delusional. Believing that normal laws and rules of human interaction don't apply to you defines mania and requires intervention. It can lead to disinhibition in behaviour: excessive spending, sexuality, rudeness and even driving. Sleep is usually affected and this is a very valuable sign. Clients may declare proudly that they 'don't need to sleep . . . it's only been two hours each night for the last week'.

The decision about whether someone is overactive because of personality, anxiety or mania is important for long-term management, but in a crisis there may be similar initial management approaches to each. Calming and competent enquiry about the client's circumstances is needed. If it is decided that this is the person's 'normal' personality, it may well be that some immediate work would be appropriate in terms of why they have ended up presenting to mental health services in crisis, but longer-term intervention would seem inappropriate. If the cause seems to be anxiety, this needs to be addressed (see Chapter 5). If mania is likely, consideration needs to be given to risk issues (see Chapter 4), medication management and problem-solving if there are specific precipitants to the manic state. Cooperation can often be achieved where good relationships exist with staff and carers but can be more difficult where they do not, or have been progressively damaged over time. Degrees of insight can persist even when someone is manic and paradoxically a client may agree to restrictions on their activities and be willing to take medication. Generally the aim is to collaborate rather than confront, but at times where potentially dangerous behaviour is involved (e.g. driving) or family members are reaching the point of exhaustion, action may need to be taken under mental health legislation.

Use of medication

Medication used in mania includes atypical anti-psychotics (e.g. Olanzepine, Quetiapine or Risperidone), which tend to be used in the acute phase supplemented with short-acting benzodiazepines where overactivity and other symptoms are causing severe disturbance. Mood stabilisers such as lithium carbonate or sodium valproate do have effects in the early stages of episodes but do not tend to be used alone in most countries, although they may be commenced in the acute phase for their later prophylactic effect. Current medication, contra-indications and side-effects, plus past experience with these drugs will affect choice.

Case example

Shirley, aged 43, had had a number of previous manic episodes so when she began to remain up for most of the night, her mother, with whom she lived, became anxious that she was becoming ill. Unfortunately this increased tension in the household, with continuing and increasingly loud arguments about Shirley going to bed. She started to stay out at night instead, her alcohol intake increased and she started a relationship with a young man she had met in the local pub. She was prepared however to meet with her mental health worker and psychiatrist and, although up and down throughout the interview and becoming increasingly flirtatious, she did concede that she might not be quite her usual self – however much she was enjoying her present lifestyle. She agreed to additional medication and increased support for herself and her mother. Over the next couple of days, tensions increased at home and she finally agreed voluntarily to come into hospital 'for a break'. Over the next month she responded fully to admission and medication.

Agitation

Agitation describes behaviour which can progress to include self-harming, overactive aggressive or anxious behaviour, but is distinct from it. Symptoms include pacing, restlessness, distress and feeling unable to sit still, and agitation has a number of causes:

- anxiety;
- depression;
- anger;
- confusion and distress from psychotic symptoms;
- side-effects from anti-psychotic and sometimes anti-depressant medication, especially 'restless legs' (akathisia);
- physical illnesses.

What can you do?

Distinction needs to be made between these different causes of agitation so that they can be individually addressed, although a number of causes may be present at the same time (e.g. anxiety and akathisia). Anxiety and depression will be accompanied by other symptoms, as described in Chapter 5. Anger will often be recognised as such by the client but not always, sometimes appearing as depression or anxiety. It will usually occur with a specific focus on a person or group of people or circumstances. However, it is sometimes only from a full assessment that it becomes clear that a grievance exists which is fuelling dissatisfaction and, ultimately, anger. Psychotic symptoms can arise from misunderstandings and a range of troublesome thoughts (see

Chapter 7) and present as agitation. Side-effects of medications can cause agitation as can a range of physical illnesses (see Chapter 8).

Some behaviour seen in crisis situations is not self-harming, overactive or aggressive but does demand attention and a response. Often the person is vocal in asking for help, either generally or specifically ('I can't go home') or is being threatening. This may be accompanied by physical demands – pushing, shoving or obstructing.

The cause of the agitation should be managed. It may be associated with physical symptoms (see Chapter 8), depression and/or anxiety (see Chapter 5) or psychotic symptoms (see Chapter 7). Calm, consistent and clear communication will help, as will distraction by discussion of neutral or positive topics. Meaningful physical activity – going out to the shops or park for example – may help.

Use of medication

Medication can assist through its sedative and anti-psychotic properties, hence sedative anti-depressants (e.g. Mirtazepine, Trazadone or Amitryptiline) and/or anti-psychotics may be appropriate. Severe agitation may warrant the use of short-term (e.g. Lorazepam) or occasionally longer-term benzodiazepines (e.g. Clonazepam). Side-effects, particularly akathisia from anti-psychotics, can exacerbate symptoms. Reduction of medication dosage is often the appropriate action to take and often reduces accompanying psychotic symptoms. If there has been a clear relationship between dose reduction and worsening of symptoms, other measures may need considering (e.g. the use of beta-blockers).

Rituals

Ritualistic behaviour can present in crisis but this is very unusual, although it may be part of a broader picture. Its causes include:

- obsessive-compulsive disorder (OCD);
- schizophrenia;
- autism;
- learning disability;
- medication side-effects;
- physical causes such as encephalitis.

What can you do?

Assessment and investigation can help establish the underlying cause. Where this is associated with troublesome thoughts (e.g. obsessions, voices or delusions), or emotional problems (e.g. depression), these need to be dealt with accordingly. However, the behaviour itself may need addressing directly with an underlying principle that because you think something you do not necessarily need to act upon it – although the nature of compulsion is that it may be difficult to resist. For obsessional rituals, developing a strategy for future management with therapeutic intervention can help to resolve the crisis by instilling hope that effective intervention is possible. The behaviour itself is often more disconcerting for the carer than the client, who may be only marginally aware of it. Understanding the carer's concern is important in working out how to cope while treatment commences. It may be that the key concern is that the behaviour is abnormal and treatment is necessary, so if it is agreed that a referral will be made, the carer may be prepared to wait for that to take effect. However, the behaviour may be a long-term problem (e.g. as part of autism), and coping methods to overcome the irritation it can cause need to be devised. Sometimes this simply means the carer taking 'time out', possibly with the support of other family members or friends, or respite being provided by statutory services.

Rituals may interfere significantly with the client's functioning and perpetuate unhappiness. Helping the client identify and recognise this may motivate them to develop ways of resisting performing the rituals where control can be exerted over them. Crisis points in their lives can sometimes enable this to happen and lead to long-term benefits.

Wandering

Occasions arise where mental health practitioners are asked to assess clients who have been found wandering and who are unable to explain what they are doing and why – even, at times, who they are. Sometimes they are able to provide a contact telephone number but not always. On other occasions they are known to services or the police, who are frequently involved in bringing them in for assessment. They may be in a fugue state, where they appear to have wandered away with accompanying loss of memory and often seem dazed and distant at interview. An amnesic syndrome may be the cause, often associated with confusion, recollections or turning up of the past and short-term confabulation (making up stories).

Causes for wandering behaviour include:

- mental health problems (such as schizophrenia), dissociative states or depression after severe trauma;
- physical disorders such as dementia and epilepsy, especially temporal lobe epilepsy, including post-ictal states (i.e. after an epileptic fit), dementia, brain injury or infection, alcohol or drug intoxication, Korsakov's psychosis (short-term memory loss from vitamin B1 deficiency, especially occurring with alcohol dependence).

What can you do?

Management involves immediate physical examination and relevant health care, for example, rehydration if needed, as self-neglect may be a feature. In relation to mental health problems, there may be significant suicide risk and this needs to be carefully assessed as the person may not appear particularly distressed. They may have experienced or witnessed significant trauma or have left behind major adverse life circumstances or events. Where no disorder is found, there usually emerges some reason to account for the behaviour when contact is eventually made with relatives and others. However, even where traumatic events have precipitated the wandering, careful assessment needs to be made that the behaviour is not an atypical presentation of dementia, depression or psychosis.

Drug and alcohol use

Drug or alcohol use frequently complicates crisis presentations and can lead to difficult management decisions. It can also carry risk to the client and others around them. This is primarily because of the disinhibiting and sedating effects of drugs and alcohol. But it can also be because of their direct effect on existing symptoms, especially depression, and can even produce new ones (e.g. paranoia and hallucinations). There are also potentially adverse effects on physical health of a chronic and acute nature. Sometimes drugs and alcohol are used in response to distress and mask diagnosis, leading to dismissal of clients who require a response from mental health teams.

Alcohol

Alcohol use is so common in society that judging whether it is relevant to a crisis is not always easy. Alcohol is popular because it is relaxing and eases social interactions for most people. Its use in home and social environments can have positive benefits. However, the nature of distress is such that alcohol is likely to increase it or at least its presentation. Alcohol is a depressant and tends to increase depression, however it is also anxiety-reducing in many instances so paradoxically may be used for reducing stress and as self-medication for symptoms such as voices or panic. Its disinhibiting effects can become damaging, leading to impulsive or aggressive behaviour. The after-effects, the 'hangover', can lead to agitation and depression and this can become longer-lasting where a withdrawal syndrome is present. Its effect on relationships and its financial cost can also exacerbate social problems.

Full assessment follows from eliciting the amount that the client has been drinking and the effects it has had.

- Recent intake (in units of alcohol); past day, past week, past few months.

- Do they think they have a problem? If so, when did drinking first became an issue (in amount or effect)?
- Pattern of drinking: binges or regular?
- Where does drinking occur – home, pub, friends' homes?
- Effects on:

  ○ behaviour: sedating, demotivating, disinhibiting, argumentative;
  ○ relationships: family, friends, partners;
  ○ finances: how much is it costing (worth working out with the client), debts;
  ○ health: correlate with past medical history (e.g. ulcers, accidents, liver problems, high blood pressure, epilepsy, neuropathy – tingling and numbness especially in legs); and current symptoms, especially abdominal pain, headaches, tremor, diarrhoea, sleep disturbance, anxiety, impotence.

- Any signs of:

  ○ withdrawal symptoms (e.g. shakes, anxiety, fearfulness, fits, craving);
  ○ delirium tremens (DTs) – as above with added confusion, visions, paranoia, insomnia, sweating, high blood pressure and pulse;
  ○ Wernicke's encephalopathy (rare but serious), staggering, flickering eye movements (nystagmus), reduced eye movements, peripheral neuropathy.

- Has the client previously sought help? Where? With what results?
- Why do they think they drink as they do?
- What do they think they need to do about it? Nothing, cut down, stop for a bit, stop for ever?
- Do they want help?

The CAGE questionnaire[6] is frequently used to detect problem drinking (yes to two or more questions may be significant):

- Have you ever felt you should *c*ut down on your drinking?
- Have people *a*nnoyed you by criticising your drinking?
- Have you ever felt bad or *g*uilty about your drinking?
- Have you ever had a drink first thing in the morning to steady your nerves or to get rid of a hangover (*e*ye opener)?

What can you do?

Incidental use of alcohol

It may be that distressing news has been imparted after the person had started drinking – they may even have been given a drink in preparation for it. The effects of alcohol will begin to diminish quickly although the amount taken will clearly influence this. It may be that deferring assessment until these effects are no longer seriously impairing the client is most appropriate. If the person is in a place of safety such as a police station or with relatives who appear to be able to contain the situation, waiting and returning later may be the best course. There are nevertheless risks with this approach which need to be weighed – risks of harm to self and others, for example.

If the situation is left, contact numbers need to be available and the time of return stated and adhered to. Consent of patient and carers should always be obtained. Occasionally if the client is detained in custody, reasons for this action may need to be given and consent may not need to be obtained. Nevertheless, agreeing a return time often helps to reduce problems.

On your return, assessment needs to proceed. It may be that underlying issues emerge which can be dealt with in the future. Assessment in itself may be very effective at working through the current crisis, problem-solving in relation to it and instilling hope. Hope for the future may be the most thera-peutic intervention offered. As the situation calms, so assessment of future care needs is possible. There may be none – sometimes simply working issues through and sobering up is all that is necessary. Sometimes it can emerge that the crisis has simply uncovered underlying issues which need further work or the cause of the crisis may have caused new problems (e.g. financial, from death of the breadwinner in the family). Not infrequently it turns out that alcohol use was not coincidental but habitual and problems with it need addressing.

Habitual use

Presentation to mental health services of someone who is habitually using alcohol or has a past history of damaging intermittent use may be clearly related to the alcohol use or not. It may be that use is denied: it may be obvious from the smell of alcohol and/or the behaviour associated that the person has been drinking but this is not always the case and it may only emerge during assessment, from blood tests or from discussion with friends and relatives, revealing that problems exist.

The presentation may be of distress or from direct effects of alcohol (e.g. a road traffic accident, leading to hospitalisation). The presenting symptoms may then be from alcohol withdrawal. In each case, there is little to be gained from immediate interview if intoxicated, once risk issues have been resolved. This depends on the circumstances and protection available (e.g. if the client is alone and homeless the decision to proceed with the interview may need to be taken sooner rather than later).

When the client is sober and can answer questions clearly and responsibly, discussion of the nature of their problems can begin. Despite a knowledge that the person has drinking problems, it makes sense to have a full initial discussion of their presenting concerns, to do as comprehensive an assessment as possible and let them tell you about their alcohol intake and issues surrounding it, if necessary with gentle prompting but with as much information as possible coming from the person themselves. It is difficult not to jump to conclusions and be judgemental but gradual eliciting of drinking behaviours can allow the person to begin to draw their own conclusions about what they need to do. Essentially a motivational interviewing approach is most likely to open up areas that the individual can take forward.

It can be helpful to consider differences in the ways in which alcohol is misused by different groups. Some individuals may have spent many years drinking as part of their occupation (e.g. if they were running a hotel or restaurant). Others, often women, who become or at least feel trapped in a relationship with no escape and feel unable to assert themselves towards others, use drink for 'Dutch courage'. Family members may seem to take advantage of their unassertiveness. Alcohol provides rapid relief of feelings of inner turmoil and may lead to them expressing themselves assertively – only to be dismissed because 'it's only the drink talking'. Finally, use of alcohol can begin young and increase in the teenage years and early 20s. It can then disinhibit already impulsive individuals. This leads to clashes with authority and subsequent rebelliousness exacerbating the situation. Eventually alcohol is left as seeming the only enjoyment, and social release and dependency leads to continuing use. Unassertive and rebellious individuals often present to services threatening to commit suicide. Past behaviour is a useful determinant of intent to do so but a careful risk assessment will be needed (see Chapter 4). Initial presentation with no previous known history or any contacts is difficult. Where there have been repeated previous episodes, with threats but no action, it is easier to decide against home treatment or admission (see Chapter 9). Many people who commit suicide do so when intoxicated and alcohol dependents are certainly at higher risk.

When a person says they are suicidal, risk assess. Discuss alternatives – do they accept they have a drink problem? Will they come back, see their family doctor or attend a counselling service in the morning to discuss available help, possibly detoxification as an inpatient or outpatient? Can they see alternatives to their current course? If they present alternatives (e.g. 'admit me or I'll kill myself'), it is unlikely (although still possible) that they are in the depths of suicidal despair. It is more likely that they want escape from a situation and possibly a bed for the night. However, admitting inappropriately can be very disruptive to other patients' care, potentially dangerous because of hostility and disinhibition, and counterproductive. A constructive interview – advice about seeking detoxification and possibly help via organisations such as Alcoholics Anonymous (AA) may be effective in some instances – more so than the easy option of admission followed by walking out the next day or discharge after continued drinking.

Often when patients present intoxicated with drugs or alcohol, they will be asking for or demanding help, and carers and friends may be reinforcing this request. Where this is the first time that the individual has accepted they need to deal with their substance problems, it can seem humane and reasonable to provide an immediate response. It is certainly important to be accepting of the client's current motivation – it may be that a window of opportunity has opened up to be exploited – but the response needs to be a considered one which has the best chance of success. Generally this is not to immediately admit to hospital or a detoxification unit as even where there is short-term abstinence, longer-term success tends to be rare. Although there is no evidence comparing immediate response to a delayed and considered one, clinical experience strongly supports asking the person to return when sober or to accept referral to a treatment service. An explanation which is frank but supportive is necessary (e.g. 'Come back tomorrow morning once the effects of alcohol have lessened and we can discuss ways we can offer you help'). If they return it suggests that they have sufficient motivation to begin to address their problems. Where such requests have occurred frequently before, a situation of diminishing returns develops – and offering detoxification becomes less and less appropriate. How then to make a decision about whether a client has actually changed? The option of suggesting they attend a certain number of AA meetings is sometimes appropriate or you could suggest they present regularly for counselling. However, AA is not for everyone; some people find groups hard or get put off by the spiritual language used. It may not be appropriate for people who have experienced sexual abuse to be in a mixed-sex group of people sharing their stories, even though they don't have to. It is an option but not the panacea for all. Older men are probably the group who find AA most helpful, especially where their social network is based around the pub and they need support to replace it.

Substance misuse services should be able to provide a reasonably rapid response to a considered request for detoxification (i.e. within days) in an ideal health system but this may not be possible with service limitations. It is worth considering in consultation with the person's family doctor whether home detoxification is possible or appropriate with assistance from other workers. However, if there have been severe withdrawal reactions in the past (e.g. convulsions), this may not be safe, although such circumstances are rare. Where delays are envisaged, advising *against* rapid reduction in alcohol use may be paradoxically appropriate, or medication can be provided.

Use of medication

In a crisis situation, medication is essentially irrelevant and can be positively dangerous. Many drugs used in these circumstances simply endanger the patient through additional sedation and possible respiratory depression where alcohol has already been consumed or is very likely to be in the near future. It may be that a home detoxification programme is appropriate but this needs to be planned with suitable supports – possibly a community team, a general practitioner and counselling, plus family and friends' involvement as appropriate, to maximise the utilisation of a window of opportunity.

Rarely patients present in a withdrawal state from alcohol and emergency treatment is then appropriate, either at home or in hospital. It may be that prescription of an anti-convulsant with benzodiazepine or alone if abstinence is not the immediate aim is appropriate. The degree of physical dependence, length of time, past history or family history of convulsions or head injury may affect this judgement. DTs is a medical emergency with a significant death rate untreated so immediate medical attention is needed. Similarly, vitamin B1 deficiency needs immediate attention as this can progress to Korsokov's psychosis which involves permanent memory loss and inability to form new memories.

The use of drugs to deter a client from drinking alcohol, such as Disulfiram ('Antabuse'), or to reduce craving (e.g. Acamprosate) is best not initiated in crisis situations even where the client has been sober, at least not without discussion with a substance misuse specialist.

Case example

Alex, aged 47, lived with a partner and her 12-year-old son, and worked as a storeman. He was found wandering in the early hours, distressed and saying that he wanted to die. He was picked up by the police and bought to the local police station where a mental health assessment was requested. He admitted drinking heavily that night. Prior to attendance, the social worker and psychiatrist who had been contacted discussed with the custody sergeant when would be reasonable to make the assessment. It was agreed that delaying the assessment until Alex was less intoxicated was appropriate and so it was made first thing the next day.

Alex was contrite and apologetic but also very low in mood. The suicidal intent of the early hours of the morning had now receded although he said the thoughts had been present for many months. He had been drinking excessively since his teens and spent most evenings in the pub or drinking at home. He had no current, or history of, physical symptoms of relevance apart from some shakiness in the morning. His partner had arrived at the police station and, whilst expressing positive feelings about how he could be, did consider his drinking to be a problem for the family.

The crisis plan involved taking a motivational interviewing approach to assessment. In discussing previous relationships and employment, Alex conceded spontaneously that alcohol had been detrimental. However, he found it very difficult to see how he could do anything about it – he said that he could cut down or stop any time if he wanted but couldn't see how this would help. He was asked about previous attempts to do this and also the relationship of his mood and social difficulties to his drinking. He admitted having tried and failed to control his drinking and recognised that alcohol had affected areas of his life. The relationship between mood and alcohol was discussed – not only in terms of its relationship to depressing events but also the direct chemical effect in depressing mood and increasing suicidality. He accepted this. The options available to him were drawn up: he could continue as he was, he could try to change things himself, he could accept help from his family doctor, a local counselling service or via referral to a substance misuse team. He decided to look for help initially from his family doctor, with whom he had discussed his drinking previously, and attend with his partner.

Communication with the family doctor and partner included a report of the assessment and options discussed with a suggestion that community detoxification be considered (using Chlordiazepoxide). Involvement of the counselling and substance misuse service would probably improve the likelihood of enduring success.

Drug misuse

Drug misuse can present in a range of ways in crisis:

* from toxic effects of overdose;
* from negative effects of the drug causing sedation, fear, distress, self-harm, physical symptoms or psychosis;
* from withdrawal effects;
* from attempts to obtain more of the drug (see Chapter 8).

Assessment, when it can be made, includes similar considerations to those for alcohol. In acute situations where the person is experiencing immediate toxic effects, establish:

* What drugs have been taken? How much? When? Past day, past week, past few months?
* How did they take the drugs? Orally, inhaled, injected?
* What were the circumstances in which they took them? Home, nightclub, friends, on streets?
* What effects have they had? Physical: sedation, arousal, accidents. Psychological: anxiety, fear, depression, hallucinations – voices, visions, being touched, paranoia.

When possible try to establish:

* whether they intend to continue taking drugs;
* how they take the drugs (HIV/hepatitis precautions, if relevant);
* whether they think they have a problem and if so when drug use first became a problem (in amount or effect);

- the pattern of drug use (binges or regular);
- where drug use occurs – home, pub, friends' homes;
- effects on: behaviour (sedating, demotivating, disinhibiting, argumentative); relationships (family, friends, partners); finances: how much it is costing (worth working out with them), debts; health, which correlate with past medical history (accidents, overdose, needle damage) and current symptoms, especially abdominal pain, headaches, tremor, diarrhoea, sleep disturbance, anxiety and impotence;
- look for signs of withdrawal symptoms.

In addition, ask the client:

- Have they previously sought help? Where? What results?
- Why do they think they use drugs as they do?
- What do they think they need to do about it?
- Do they want help?

What can you do?

Generally mental health practitioners do not become involved directly in responses to overdose but may be called to assess later. However, they often see negative psychological effects presenting in crisis and management can be difficult. Often the person themselves or others with them will disclose that they have taken an illicit drug but the amount or even type can be vague and unclear. Further assessment can be very difficult and, as with alcohol, awaiting recovery from the effects of intoxication is necessary. However, risk issues need to be assessed as risk to self or to others can be significant (e.g. from responding to hallucinations and paranoia). In general, quiet, calm surroundings with familiar people who can reassure and protect the client from themselves are ideal. Police stations and hospitals rarely meet these environmental criteria but nevertheless can provide safety while the effects of the drugs wear off. Usually the reduction in the acute effect happens quite quickly with improvements occurring in two or three hours (although this does depend on the amount and strength of the compound involved) and most signs gone within 8–12 hours, leaving a fairly exhausted and sometimes still anxious individual.

Solvent abuse can present, especially in adolescents, with agitation, restlessness or drowsiness, glazed expression, slurred speech and clumsy gait. Sometimes this is accompanied by a red rash around the mouth from the direct effect of the solvent on the skin. Heavy use has been known to cause asphyxia (interference with breathing especially from the plastic bags sometimes used), heart irregularities (arrythmias), injury and even death.

Hallucinogenic drugs, such as LSD, amphetamines, cocaine and cannabis (especially where this is particularly potent), can precipitate psychotic episodes which are indistinguishable from schizophrenia or hypomania. Cocaine can also present with marked affective instability – mood fluctuation – and tactile hallucinations. They can be distinguished by absence of previous such symptoms prior to taking the drug and will wear off as the effects of the drug reduce. Urine testing can establish presence of these drugs with kits available in most acute units and police stations allowing immediate results. Where recovery is rapid and full, no further action is needed although it may be worth involving early intervention services to provide support for a period, as sometimes the consequence of such episodes is recurrence – certainly anyone presenting in this way is at increased risk of developing a longer-term problem, not necessarily psychosis; panic, PTSD-like symptoms, depersonalisation syndrome and depression are all possible.

However, things are often not as straightforward to diagnose; it may be that the person has used drugs regularly in the past but never had such a negative reaction, or they have had emerging or definite symptoms prior to the drug use and this may be precipitating a longer-term problem. It is as well to have a high index of suspicion and provide follow-up and contact numbers after recovery has occurred. If recovery is not occurring within a few hours or some symptoms (e.g. paranoia or hallucinations) are persisting, intensive home treatment or admission to hospital needs to be considered.

Withdrawal states are relevant for opiates in particular. Cocaine, amphetamines, LSD and cannabis generally do not cause physical dependence although users may describe psychological symptoms. Opiate withdrawal presents with agitation, fearfulness, nausea and vomiting, abdominal and muscle cramps, shivering, dilated pupils, tearfulness, sweating and runny nose (rhinorrhea). It is not a life-threatening condition but needs medical attention. It is very unpleasant and treatment includes use of Naltrexone, Methodone and benzodiazepines. Benzodiazepines, if stopped abruptly, can cause a withdrawal syndrome with tingling, ears ringing (tinnitus), giddiness (vertigo), hypersensitivity to sounds (hyperacusis), confusion and, very rarely, seizures.

It is necessary to notify the chief medical officer of anyone presenting with addiction to illegal drugs. This may seem contrary to developing a good relationship and a breach of confidentiality but is a statutory requirement. Telling the client this – which they may already know – can reduce their negative reaction to it happening.

Longer-term support to assist with drug problems will usually be provided by substance misuse services (including non-statutory advisory agencies) and links can be made with them at this time. As discussed in Chapter 1, crisis can be a time for renewal and moving forward and this is particularly the case with addictive behaviours. The individual can reach a turning point at which appreciation of the nature of their problems occurs and a belief that change is possible converts into action and hope for the future.

Compulsive behaviours

Presentation as a consequence of compulsive behaviour such as gambling, some rituals (see above) and some substance misuse (see above) occurs occasionally in crisis – usually where others have found out that this has become a problem for the person and the consequences may have become a problem for the family unit as a whole. Alternatively, the person may present with depression as part of a manic picture or may simply be demanding help. Occasionally depression can lead to gambling through its effects on judgement and the feelings of hopelessness or vulnerability to others it generates, and if it appears that depression preceded the gambling behaviour, treatment of the depression alone may help, although the financial and relationship consequences may need to be repaired. Mania and disinhibition can lead to reckless behaviour including gambling, and again treatment of the illness and its consequences is the way forward.

Where, as is most common, the gambling is the cause rather than result of a person's problems, assessment of how compulsive the behaviour has become and development of a management plan to overcome it is the right approach.

What can you do?

In relation to gambling, there is not a great deal that mental health practitioners can do as there is currently little evidence for effectiveness and even less for availability of psychological services to provide assistance (with the exception of some individual psychologists with a special interest). There is potential for providing justification for behaviour inadvertently which can mean that the client does not take action themselves and any carer becomes confused about responsibility issues. However, some immediate planning of how to manage the consequences of behaviour and limit future damage may be possible. Self-help groups such as Gamblers Anonymous can provide a route for support.

Demanding behaviour

Behaviour where the client or their carer is energetically asking for assistance is a very common presentation. Initially, responses from practitioners are often to assume this is not due to mental health problems but 'behavioural' or due to personality issues. However, such behaviour can be the presentation of someone who is:

• distressed;
• confused;
• frightened;

- in pain;
- used to having to demand to gain attention;
- frustrated with their current situation.

It is therefore important to fully assess and on that basis manage any underlying mental health problems. If none can be detected, the situation should be managed in a way to reduce risk and distress to all concerned. It is also important to express any doubts that are relevant and provide contact telephone numbers in the event that matters change. There are some indicators which suggest that the behaviour is not due to mental disorder and therefore mental health service intervention is not appropriate. For example, the client is:

- trying to make others including the practitioner feel responsible for their actions;
- found to be withholding information which seems to be for their own gain (rather than because of its intimate or otherwise private or distressing nature);
- found to be deceiving or fabricating statements or has a history of doing so (although people can fabricate because their experience is such that this is the only way of getting their feelings of distress validated);
- particularly resistant and uncooperative (not related to psychosis or depression);
- expressing resentment towards others;
- avoiding difficult circumstances or otherwise gaining or likely to gain from the current assessment or management (e.g. through admission to hospital – see Chapter 8).

Box 6.1 Behaviour checklist

- Consider:

  - Is the behaviour a presenting symptom of a mental health problem such as depression, OCD, autism, substance misuse, anxiety, mania or schizophrenia?
  - Are there positive reasons for considering personality issues, especially long-standing relationship problems? What type? Borderline, dependent, antisocial, obsessional or schizoid?
  - Are both personality issues and mental health problems present?

- Self-harm:

  - deal with immediate consequences;

- o   assess continuing risk and develop management of this;
- o   try to empathise with distress and reasons for self-harm;
- o   begin planning for support and alternative ways of coping.

- Aggression:

  - o   immediate focus on safety;
  - o   de-escalate situation;
  - o   enquire into reasons for aggression; problem-solve if appropriate;
  - o   consider if medication has a role.

- Agitation:

  - o   consider mental health problem;
  - o   review reasons and treat accordingly;
  - o   consider effects of medication.

- Overactivity:

  - o   assess reasons;
  - o   assess risks;
  - o   manage any mental health problem;
  - o   try to collaborate and draw on insight;
  - o   consider use of medication.

- Substance misuse:

  - o   assess risks;
  - o   wait until intoxication is wearing off before assessing if possible;
  - o   assess level of dependence/interference in life;
  - o   use motivational interviewing style;
  - o   assess motivation for help: set up if responsive, with family doctor or substance misuse counselling/team;
  - o   consider appropriate support/advice for carers.

- Compulsive behaviours:

  - o   manage as part of any mental health problem;
  - o   gambling: assess if consequent on depression, mania, etc., set out plan to manage financial and relationship consequences, consider Gamblers Anonymous.

Perspectives from a group of clients

Generally [the chapter] is felt to explain and give good advice on [among other things] why people self-harm and how to deal with this. It could mention some common unhelpful responses people have encountered, i.e. 'Pull yourself together and you can have a nice suit like mine', said by a psychiatrist in accident and emergency to a male who had cut his arms (!). Most group members have felt that their medication (usually anti-depressants) has been helpful in managing their feelings that lead to self-harm. The gender of the person treating self-harm was felt to be unimportant by people in the group. Individual attitude and empathy were felt to be more important.

We felt that the paragraph on crisis planning and providing follow-up measures after repeated crises on p. 127 to be very important – where this has happened this has been extremely helpful, however repeated self-harm has usually met with a negative response.

The group would like to stress that people self-harm when they feel that they cannot express/alleviate their distress in any other way – therefore self-harm is a coping strategy that works for them. It is unrealistic and unhelpful to expect/demand that this behaviour stops without help to investigate alternative coping strategies. Dealing with self-harm in a punitive way often causes further distress, leading to further self-harm and avoidance of services/support in future.

Penny and the Bedford House Self Harm Support Group

Troublesome thoughts

There are a variety of thoughts which can present as distressing in crisis:

- depressive;
- hypochondriacal;
- suicidal;
- delusional;
- hallucinatory, especially voices and visions;
- thought disorder
- obsessional;
- feelings of unreality (depersonalised and derealised);
- confusion;
- even 'normal' thoughts.

These accompany distressed mood and behaviour frequently and each needs to be focused upon in its own right (see Chapter 5 for discussion of depressive thoughts, Chapter 8 for hypochondriacal thoughts and Chapter 6 for behavioural presentations). Often these thoughts need addressing directly. We will start with a discussion of 'normal thinking' before moving on to discuss the other types of thoughts that can present.

'Normal' thinking

Sometimes people present in crisis because of a fear that their thinking is abnormal, that they are going mad or are evil. This can accompany:

- anxiety and be managed accordingly (see Chapter 5);
- an exacerbation of depressive symptoms (e.g. thinking transiently of suicide which may be considered evil because of religious belief or family responsibilities);
- obsessional symptoms which can also be a response to depression and represent overconcern and reading meaning into something inappropriately;

- misunderstanding of 'automatic thoughts' and how they flow on regardlessly can be concerning at times;
- transient hallucinations, especially related to bereavement or other traumatic experiences, can distress. Various non-pathological perceptions which may be misunderstood as hallucinations are possible also which can cause worry. For examples, 'eidetic' images involving voluntary recall of a remembered object or scene; retinal after-images and pareidolia – images provoked by abstract sensory impressions (e.g. seeing people's heads in clouds).

Overcoming the crisis involves attempting to 'normalise' the situation by explaining that:

- the client's thoughts are not abnormal;
- they need not worry directly about them;
- their thoughts do not imply that they are going mad or are evil;
- they can move on to dealing with day-to-day issues in their life;
- thoughts and actions are distinct – because they think something doesn't mean they are bad, mad or need to act upon it.

Insight involves identification of abnormality and an awareness of this. Explaining that the person's awareness of the problems, even where this is simply worry about normal phenomena, is a sign that they are not 'going mad'.

Suicidal thoughts

These are discussed under risk management (Chapter 4) and in the management of depression (Chapter 5) but they can become an issue in their own right. As described above under 'normal' thoughts, suicidal thoughts accompanying a brief distressing or depressive episode, or even moment, can in turn lead to negative thoughts about the client themselves, such as, 'There must be something wrong with me' or 'I must be evil or ungrateful to think that'. This can become distressing and disturbing in its own right. It is important to assess associated risk but if the client is clearly of low risk and has no intent or plans to act on the thoughts, discussing how common such thoughts are will help. General population surveys have demonstrated one in ten of the population in any two-week period will have experienced such thoughts. It is also reasonable to explain such thoughts as being a response to a negative emotion – an automatic thought – which corresponds to a wish not to feel that way. This can express itself as a wish to escape from that feeling and a suicidal thought may be a natural response. But if the client does not wish to act upon it – as they have stated they don't – there is no reason for them to do so and they can move on.

Where suicidal thoughts are linked to intent and distress, a risk management plan needs to be drawn up (see Chapter 3) but it may also be necessary to discuss the thoughts themselves. While some of this work can be done following the immediate crisis, sometimes discussion is necessary to defuse the crisis and it can be therapeutic to do so. Directive statements are usually not helpful but working out a balanced consideration may be, with reasons for and against (in that order). Where circumstances are particularly adverse this can be difficult (e.g. after the death of a partner or the diagnosis of a terminal illness). Finding out what the particular fears are (e.g. loneliness, pain, loss of status) can allow you to address these directly. Relationships often feature high on the list of reasons against but absence or breakdown in them can be major reasons for, from the client's point of view. Spiritual beliefs may protect as can enlisting the help of relatives. Sometimes, however, you are only left with the proposition that time can be a healer, alongside mental health interventions, and trying to instil hope that things can get better.

Delusional thoughts

When somebody presents in crisis saying things that seem to make no sense, it is easy to jump to the conclusion that they are deluded. It is very important not to – even if it emerges that they have beliefs that meet criteria for delusions. Reaching such a conclusion without exploring the beliefs with the person can be profoundly damaging to the relationship you develop with them – at that time, during the initial interview and in the future.

People will express strange things for a variety of reasons:

- because they are true;
- because they are partially true but misunderstood, exaggerated or got out of context;
- because they have misunderstood things said or expressed in other ways;
- because their manner of expressing themselves is not good – they mean something else; they may use phrases or words inaccurately, thinking they mean something different;
- because they are teasing or humouring you;
- because they are testing out your reaction;
- because it is their way of handling anxiety (talking nonsense or gibberish);
- because there is an underlying neurological reason (e.g. from dysphasia caused by damage to the brain incurred by a stroke or tumour);
- because they believe something that is not true in a strictly logical or scientific sense but is culturally appropriate; or may be a reasonable response to their own previous personal experiences; or is very difficult to understand even with knowledge of the person's background.

Delusions are strong beliefs that can have a wide variety of themes:

- paranoia;
- ideas of delusions of reference (e.g. from other people or sources of sound such as radio, TV or music);
- grandiosity;
- thought interference (being read, broadcast, inserted or taken out of the mind);
- beliefs in infidelity of partner (morbid jealousy);
- infatuation with another person which is not reciprocated (erotomania);
- belief in the replacement of a relative or friend by a double (Capgras syndrome);
- infestation with parasites, having disease or bodily change that doesn't exist (monosymptomatic hypochondriacal psychosis).

Delusions may be presenting symptoms or emerge as aspects of a problem which may present as a social or relationship crisis. There may be variation in how strongly the beliefs are held and sometimes they can change with brief discussion. Those that cause most concern and distress are those which are held strongly and seem fixed and to be seriously interfering with the client's or other people's lives.

What can you do?

Identifying relevant issues is covered in Chapter 2. A key issue is the importance of a broad approach, not just a blinkered one to symptoms excluding key precipitants. It is also very important to view any crisis in this situation as part of an actual or potentially long-term problem, the outcome of which can be affected very significantly by the actions taken in this crisis. Time expended on developing cooperation and avoiding or minimising compulsory measures can potentially save or at least minimise years of distress and disability and the need for treatment in the future.

The client may be presenting for the first time or with a relapse or worsening of symptoms. Early intervention (see Chapter 9) is important in each instance to reduce the impact of the initial episode and relapse or worsening – the longer the symptoms go without a response the more damage can occur, some of which can be difficult or even impossible to repair (e.g. job loss because of paranoid or erratic behaviour at work). The way in which the psychotic episode is managed can affect the damage it causes and how traumatic it is to the client. This in turn can have effects on future collaboration over medication and psychosocial management and also the persistence and worsening of symptoms themselves. PTSD related to acute admission to hospital has been described although the full blown syndrome is probably not common.

The principles regarding engagement (see Chapter 2) apply and skilled application of them is a key element and possibly the most therapeutic component of all. If a relationship in which mutual respect and trust exists, or can be developed rapidly, this counteracts paranoia and anxiety, and the intensity and distress of hallucinations, which may moderate the behaviour associated with delusional beliefs. It can also mean that involuntary measures can be avoided or used with least compulsion, which again can reduce the potential long-term damage.

Exacerbation or precipitation of psychotic symptoms is usually a response to life events and circumstances – although occasionally, such as with persistent voices, it is because of the cumulative attrition from their distressing effect. Identifying triggers is useful and worth exploring at crisis times, even if the level of symptoms makes it difficult.

Whatever the circumstances, trying to understand why the person says what they say is essential. Straightforward questioning can help uncover relevant material. For example:

- What makes you think that happened?
- Why do think you would want to do that?
- When did you first believe that?

Such gentle questioning is valuable as beliefs can sometimes be perpetuated by circumstances, especially paranoid beliefs. If the person is able to discuss the circumstances surrounding the first time these thoughts occurred, this can clarify where the beliefs originated from and can be very helpful in cementing a relationship.

In a crisis, there are two main considerations:

- Is the person distressed by the beliefs?
- Will they act on them?

Distress may be because of the feared consequences of the beliefs (e.g. feeling paranoid is by its nature unpleasant, anxiety- and sometimes anger-provoking and can be very depressing). Exploration and explanation can be immediately helpful. Simply being able to share the experience and get someone else's perspective on it can help – assuming an adequate relationship, the client may be prepared to accept that whatever the long-term consequences of their beliefs, in the short term, possibly because of support at home or in hospital, they are going to be safe. The fact that they have disclosed their concerns may make them feel that now that somebody knows, the feared perpetrators are less likely to act, although the reverse is also possible. Additionally, the development of ways of coping with the beliefs may reduce distress.

Behaviour in response to the beliefs needs to be considered in terms of risk (see Chapter 4) and interference with the client's own and others' lives. If their beliefs are not distressing (e.g. grandiose) this may lead to ill-judged actions which could endanger themselves or others, or their relationships, reputation or financial position. Discussion of these potential effects is worthwhile although may be refuted by the person. Despite such expressions, patients do nevertheless sometimes change behaviour in the short- or long-term.

Sometimes underlying beliefs emerge in crisis which are relevant to the delusions (e.g. 'I've always felt inferior'), and where these do surface, focusing discussion upon them rather than the delusional material can move the discussion on to more fruitful topics for future work: 'I may not be able to agree with you that you are the Lord of the Isles but this feeling of being inferior is distressing and we can certainly work on that or I can get you help for you to do so.'

Agreement to differ is a useful strategy where discussion of beliefs is becoming interminable and going round in circles; 'OK – I don't think we are going to agree on this although I'm beginning to understand why you believe it.'

A care plan is then needed to resolve the crisis. This may occasionally include compulsory measures where significant risk of serious harm exists but can often be done with a minimum of 'bad feeling' when time has been taken to explore relevant issues (see Chapter 3).

The care plan will build on the problems identified at assessment, provided the person is prepared to work with them. Where collaboration is proving difficult, it may be possible to agree that, even if the client doesn't believe they have any problems themselves, they have a problem with other people because their family or others think they are not well. Ask the client:

- Why do you think this is?
- What can we do about it?
- Do we need to work out a way of explaining to your family that you just want to be left alone?

Such an approach can allow you to get alongside the person as an ally rather than a foe. It may mean that you need to take responsibility from the family for monitoring the person's health and safety – and that involves gaining their trust and respect. This can be reinforced if you can negotiate with the person a reasonably frequent way of keeping them informed.

Positive symptoms can seem damaging and frightening but it is negative symptoms – especially low motivation – that are most disabling, although these don't tend to be presenting symptoms in crises. Keeping a balance is essential – medication may dull the voices or the paranoia but the resulting sedation may reduce drive so that the person becomes isolated and withdrawn, and increasingly hopeless. Many people function very effectively even while experiencing high levels of paranoia, hallucinations or even grandiosity – beliefs and behaviour can seem to be contradictory.

Finally, it is important to consider what carers might be able to do. Engagement is needed with the family: communication about what you think the problem is, what you are doing about it and why. The client may be doing 'odd' things and there may be pressures from neighbours for explanation or swift resolution. Discussion about precisely why the behaviour is problematic can identify new ways of coping. Practitioners often ask the family to back off and allow the client space but the result can be the client not eating, drinking or seeing anyone, and feeling angry and frightened. Responsibility for monitoring needs to be agreed with the carer and ways to make contact established if certain things happen or progress is not occurring.

Case example

Doreen, aged 57, lived with her husband, had no children and little family contact. She presented distressed, hearing voices and with paranoia of onset over a period of about two weeks. This had come on following her husband returning home after being in hospital having had a heart attack from which he had made a full recovery. She had been very worried about him and been sleeping poorly.

She was seen at home at her family doctor's and husband's request because she was refusing to leave the house. She described the voices as being from the devil, telling her she was evil and that her neighbours were going to kill her. She had already refused medication and hospitalisation as she could see no reason for these.

A simple formulation of her problems drew links between concern about her husband's illness because of her good and dependent relationship with him and consequent lack of sleep. This in turn made her vulnerable to hearing voices and she had become over-sensitive to a perceived threat from her neighbours.

The crisis plan involved work with the voices and beliefs: trying to make sense of them in context, 'normalising' them in terms of stress and sleep problems and discussing the development of the beliefs about the neighbours. Use of anti-psychotic medication was clearly indicated and hospitalisation or additional support was considered.

Doreen engaged with the discussion about the voices and beliefs well and described how her neighbours, who were quite new in the area, had been rather cold towards her when she spoke to them. She continued to hold strongly to her paranoid beliefs, to refuse medication and hospitalisation. She was not threatening the neighbours so it was agreed to involve the home treatment team and see whether it was possible over a few days to persuade her to start medication. Doreen's husband was keen to try this route at least initially, despite the nature of his health problems. Eventually Doreen did require admission to hospital, involuntarily after erratic and infrequent taking of medication, persistent distress and concerns about the effects on her husband's health. But she went calmly (complaining of it being 'unillegal', a neologism meaning completely illegal) and when there, accepted medication and continued discussion of her beliefs and voices to good effect.

Box 7.1 Delusions checklist

- Assess nature, conviction and level of interference with life.
- Consider risk issues.
- When did the client first get these thoughts?
- How have they developed?
- What has brought them to prominence now?
- What evidence supports them?
- What evidence is against them? Any alternative explanations?
- Is there any immediate way of testing them out?
- Agree to differ if necessary for treatment, increased support or hospitalisation to occur.
- Consider use of medication.
- Discuss possibilities of longer-term cognitive behaviour therapy work to explore beliefs further.

Voices

Assessment involves understanding levels of distress, frequency, preoccupation, interference with daily life, what the voices are saying, if the client recognises the voice or voices and establishing their beliefs about the voices. For example, where do they believe the voices come from? Who or what do they think causes them?

What can you do?

When the client says that the major problem is voices, increased medication is an obvious route to take but improving understanding and empowerment may be an even more effective way of helping them. It can be helpful – even in a crisis – to clarify beliefs about the origins of the voice or voices. Checking that the voices they hear are like 'you or me speaking' can be helpful in establishing that you understand the intensity and 'reality' of the experience. Asking whether others hear the voices can establish the client's understanding of their nature: that the voices are a unique experience to them. They may be unclear about this, especially if they have been isolated or the voices are new to them. You can ask them to tell you when they hear the voices and compare experiences. Sometimes 'voices' are actually misinterpretations of sounds (e.g. the hum of a refrigerator, or mumbled sounds, even clear speech, from outside the room the client is in. When voices are not occurring while you are with the client, you can ask them to try to record their experience on a tape-recorder later and then discuss it after the crisis is over.

Most patients are already aware that others can't hear the voices. Asking the client why they think others can't hear the voices allows them to reflect on the 'strangeness' of the experience and may lead to explanations which aid understanding. The client may attribute the voices to God or the devil, or believe that it is the neighbours or MI5. Or they may say that the voices are due to 'my illness' or 'schizophrenia', or they may simply not know. Discussion of ways that stress can lead to voices when someone is vulnerable, or an analogy with dreaming can be helpful – explain that voices are effectively 'dreaming awake'.

In itself, such 'normalising' can have a potent effect – it begins to make disturbing experiences understandable. It can also make the client feel less different – just because they hear voices they are not a different kind of person as they sometimes feel or are made to feel by others. It can reduce the fear that they are 'going mad'. Madness can be explained as being much more than simply the experience of voices or paranoia, but requiring beliefs about these experiences being caused by others. That they can be caused by the stress a client is under when they are particularly vulnerable can be much more acceptable. In itself this can sometimes reduce stress and anxiety, in turn having a direct effect on the voices and other symptoms.

Such understanding may also help with issues about control of the voices: if it is to do with me, the client can argue, my illness or the stress I'm under, it means that doing something myself about the stress or the experience (e.g. through medication use) may help. It may also influence beliefs about whether the voices are speaking the truth or not as they may be based on my previous experiences or be a result of my mood (usually anxious, depressed and confused).

Talking about the content of the voices can help but needs to be done cautiously and collaboratively. Asking what the voices are saying directly may be too much for the client. Asking if they think they can talk about what the voices are saying is gentler and more likely to be successful. If yes, they may still only be able to tell you the general nature of what is said where the content is abusive or derogatory. Sometimes voices are not negative or neutral and this will be easier for the person to discuss. If they feel unable to talk at all about the voices, reinforcing that that is OK, and suggesting that it may be because what the voices say is too distressing to describe is helpful. The client can also be told that sometimes voices will tell them not to talk to others, especially mental health staff.

It may still be possible and helpful to talk a bit about the voices in a relatively detached and impersonal way. For example, saying that you quite often meet people who are hearing voices, which can be a very unpleasant experience (where you think this is the case for them), may allow you to discuss ways of managing them.

If the client is able to discuss the content of voices, even in crisis it can be worth considering what is being said. It may be nonsensical, a spontaneous flow of thoughts, and is usually then not particularly distressing and can be normalised. Implications can be discussed, for example, whether the voices or discussion or response to them is impairing social relationships (e.g. walking down the road speaking out loud may look strange (unless you are holding a mobile phone to your ear)). Voices are more often distressing than pleasant and consist of specific statements which are abusive or commanding. Eliciting what these are, what they mean to the person and then assessing their validity or otherwise can be worthwhile. It can be useful to start off by asking the client why they think these things are being said to them – they may give you a very specific reason which you can then discuss. Usually they are not clear but may link it with previous events (e.g. assaults, abuse or bullying). Discussion of the relevance of those precipitating events to current circumstances can help.

Taking specific statements may be worthwhile. For example, the voices say 'you're ****ing useless': what are the things about you that support this statement? What is there against it? Weighing up the pros and cons can begin to undermine the acceptance of the statement as true and therefore warranted. It can then be possible to develop a specific way of responding to the voices (e.g. 'I'm OK – tell me why you think I'm not'). Other coping strategies may also be helpful, such as relaxation and social contact (see Box 7.2). Getting angry or pleading with the voices doesn't work for most clients although some may have found ways of exerting influence by, for example, swearing back at them, or firmly and briefly talking to them – in private.

The voices may be commanding and this can be particularly disturbing. Often clients simply accept without question that they must obey what the voices say although their actions are usually inconsistent with this, with them only acting on lesser commands rather than those which involve serious harm to self or others. However, the latter can happen, particularly with self-harming actions. Discussing the reasons for the client's belief can follow work on understanding where the voices come from. Often the belief is because of the way the voices have arisen or their loud and insistent quality, and this can be discussed: 'Because they shout at you doesn't mean you have to do what they say any more than if I shouted at you.'

Often the voices will continue to be loud and unpleasant until the client acts on them and sometimes not even then. Work with coping, including use of medication and responding can help. Accepting their existence while not acting on their commands, but not fighting them may be an approach worth exploring – the calmer and less agitated the client becomes the less insistent the voices.

> **Box 7.2 Coping strategies with voices**
>
> - *Behavioural control*: e.g. taking a warm bath, going for walk or other exercise, using a relaxation tape, using a tape, CD or MP3 player playing classical or rock music, retreat to a quiet place.
> - *Socialisation*: e.g. friends, clubs, day centres.
> - *Mental health care*: e.g. use medication, call mental health worker.
> - *Cognitive control*: such as distraction, e.g. playing a videogame, watching TV, listening to music, doing crosswords, meditation, prayer, a mantra or humming to self. Focusing and accepting, e.g. let the voice be and relax.
> - *Rational responding*: to the voice content using anxiety or anger reducing responses or do something to bring the voices on (to demonstrate controllability), give the voices a ten-minute slot at a specified time in the day. Use normalising explanations, e.g. explain it as 'schizophrenia playing up'. Combat the seemingly 'all knowing, all powerful' nature of voices; voices are not actions and need not lead to them. Begin to be assertive with the voices by developing a dialogue with them.

Case example

Jenny, aged 29, single and living alone, presented in extreme distress to accident and emergency having taken a small overdose of anti-psychotics. She eventually admitted that she was hearing voices which were very abusive to her and were telling her to kill herself. She had experienced these intermittently over the past 20 years but only recently following the breakdown of a relationship had they become so prominent.

During the assessment it became clear that there had been incidents in her childhood prior to the onset of the voices which were relevant to them. However, Jenny didn't yet feel able to discuss these. She still had contact with her mother intermittently and one or two close female friends.

The crisis plan focused on working out ways to understand and cope with the voices. It was agreed that they were male and sounded like someone shouting abuse at her. However, she readily accepted that the voices were not audible to others and that they might have something to do with past events. A very brief explanation of how voices can develop in response to stress was given. The issue was how to cope with them and reduce their intensity. Her current coping strategies were discussed and a few more (e.g. various forms of relaxation), were to be tried in the future.

Statements made by the voices were debated and refuted: she was not an evil person nor did she have to kill herself. Various reasons why she did not want to die were rehearsed. Ways of responding to the voices were explored. Showing that there were ways of working to cope with the voices and the underlying distress that Jenny felt was important in instilling hope for the future and referral for support and longer-term work was agreed. A self-help 'voices' group at a local day centre was also mentioned as a possible support and contact details were given.

Medication was also discussed: it had had some limited effect so far and it was agreed that a modest increase, taken consistently, might help, and that at the doses prescribed, was unlikely to cause any harmful side-effects.

Box 7.3 Voices checklist

- Assess nature and beliefs about the voices
- Discuss nature of the phenomena: 'Is it like someone speaking to you as I'm doing now?'
- Explore individual nature of perception: can anybody else hear the the voices? Could the client tape-record them?
- Explore the client's beliefs about the origin of the voices. Why do they think other people can't hear them?
- Explore any doubts that emerge from these discussions.
- Look for explanations, e.g. schizophrenia, and explain the nature of such conditions to the client.
- Use normalising explanations, e.g. deprivation states and other stressful circumstances, such as bereavement or PTSD.
- Encourage the client to come to the conclusion that the voices are in fact their own thoughts.
- If the client still believes the voices to belong to others, link this with the analogy of waking dreams or 'living nightmares'. Other explanations may include emotionally-charged memories (events or traumas that are etched onto the memory and are easily recalled or triggered); deprivation states; 'normal' hallucinations.
- Explore other people's experiences of the same phenomena, demonstrating that the client's condition is not unique; they are not alone.
- Discuss the client's coping strategies and suggest others.
- Use rational responding, e.g. 'I don't accept what you say because . . .'
- Discuss the client's beliefs about the need to do what the voices tell them.
- Allow the client to discuss any related trauma, if they wish to.

Thought disorder

Thought disorder can interrupt assessment and is probably most usefully viewed as a difficulty in communication rather than a disorder of thoughts in itself. It may present as unusual words or difficult to follow sentences which relate to the concepts that the person wants to describe but are inexact. Sometimes patients will use words inappropriately – thinking they mean something different – or they will fire off sentences without fully concentrating on the sequence of words they are saying. They may sometimes use metaphor or words with individual meaning to them or simply make up hybrid words. In these circumstances there is a balance between engagement and clarification that needs to be maintained. Initially allowing the client to express themselves for a short period can be necessary to establish a relationship. This done, then begin to question the client or feed back your understanding or misunderstanding of what they are saying. If the client says things which are barely intelligible or unintelligible for too long this can lead to frustration for them. They may be expecting you to understand and consequently become very frustrated when you don't, which can be interpreted as your humouring them. Often there are themes within the conversation which become apparent and focusing the conversation on these can be effective in improving mutual understanding. At times, when emotionally distressing events are discussed or the person feels pressured for other reasons, the thought disorder can become worse so there is a need to regulate the pace and depth of discussion to maintain contact with the client.

Using medication for psychotic symptoms

Medication usually has a part to play but jumping to a medication solution too quickly can make the situation worse. Time discussing symptoms and precipitants frequently reduces agitation, improves understanding and allows the relationship to develop such that collaboration rather than compulsion is possible. The amount of medication used can be reduced and is less likely to cause adverse effects which can cause difficulties with management regimes in the future.

Occasionally the symptoms are so distressing that an immediate medical solution needs to be offered: anti-psychotics, especially sedative ones, may provide short-term relief. Short-term IM injections may be necessary in an emergency with longer-acting compounds used (e.g. Zuclopenthixol acetate) where the acute symptoms seem likely to take days to resolve. Benzodiazepines are more immediate – Lorazepam is often used in these circumstances because of its rapid action – minutes rather than hours. Intramuscular use will be faster but not greatly so and the disruption involved in providing medication by this means may outweigh the benefit of slightly faster action.

More gradual exacerbation or precipitation of symptoms may also need a medical approach – a change of medication or increased dosage. If the person is only on a low dose of an anti-psychotic drug, discussion of whether they would like to increase the dose and see if that helps is sensible. The amount of the increase is be determined by the degree of distress and the nature of other interventions available. If there is a clear psychosocial intervention that is relevant, increasing the dose need only be short term, or may not be necessary at all. Discussion of alternatives is respectful, empowering and more likely to lead to agreed action (see Chapter 3 on collaboration). It is important to discuss and not downplay possible adverse effects (e.g. side-effects or family opinion where this is hostile to medication use). It is certainly important to suggest that the dosage is reviewed soon to see if it has been beneficial and whether it needs to remain at an increased level. The dose may need to be increased further but often can be reduced to previous levels which allows for transient increases in the future if necessary. Medication can easily creep up over time and then when crisis arises there is little latitude for a further increase because of the side-effects. It could be argued that higher levels might prevent relapse in the first place but, equally, high levels increase adverse effects (e.g. akathisia which can present as agitation and sedation which can lead to impaired coping with social circumstances and therefore increased social crises).

Where medication levels are already substantial (e.g. at or near maximum recommended levels), it can still be tempting to increase further but this is rarely helpful. Often it increases symptoms because of side-effects, akathisia and sedation as mentioned above. Reducing medication may seem paradoxical but patients will sometimes be quite prepared to accept this if the intention is to improve their functioning, reduce their side-effects and even increase motivation and coping abilities. Where Diazepam or other benzodiazepines are being used, explanation of the negative effects these have on mood and self-perception (see Chapter 5) can also lead to the commencement of a withdrawal programme and improved morale.

Adding new medication may be an option. Certainly if the patient is depressed or very anxious an anti-depressant may be worthwhile. If the client is already taking an anti-depressant the dose can be increased to therapeutic levels. Adding a second anti-psychotic is difficult to justify and more likely to cause complications than improve symptoms. A mood stabiliser such as Carbamazepine may be considered. Sodium valproate or lithium can be used; these help to manage manic symptoms where these are the presenting problem or where grandiosity and overactivity are major components of the clinical picture. Different preparations of medication can be worth considering (e.g. rapidly dispersible, liquid or injectable depot).

Whether changing medication is useful depends on the presenting picture. In the longer term, initiation of Clozapine may be appropriate where symptoms are not responding. Describing such a change with the hope that it can give future improvement/relief can be an appropriate intervention in crisis. Telling the client that a third of people with persistent symptoms taking Clozapine show major improvement should instil hope. In terms of effect, changing from one anti-psychotic to another is unlikely to make much positive difference as there is little good quality evidence of differential effects (apart from Clozapine as discussed). It can be quite disruptive and establishing an appropriate equivalent dose takes time, during which deterioration can occur. It may be worth changing an anti-psychotic where side-effects or additional effects are an issue. A more sedative anti-psychotic may be reasonable to offer (e.g. Olanzepine or Quetiapine) where agitation or sleep disturbance are problematic. Conversely, where sedation is interfering with functioning or causing paradoxical distress ('I feel woozy all the time'; 'I don't feel in control'; 'I've got no motivation') it may be worth changing to a *less* sedative drug (e.g. Aripiprazole). However, changing medication during a crisis period needs to be very carefully considered and only performed where there is a clear gain expected. Changing anti-depressant for similar reasons may be considered with similar provisos.

There is always a temptation to increase medication so that you are offering *something*. It is a temptation that needs resisting if better alternatives – often non-pharmacological – are available. But occasionally where something might just help – and is described to the patient frankly as such – medication tinkering can invoke placebo effects to some benefit. This is often done in practice although ethically dubious unless explained to the patient: 'There isn't much/any evidence that increasing medication will help, we need to consider the possible adverse effects, but if you are willing to accept an increase, we can offer that and see whether any benefit results. If not or the negative effects outweigh the positive, we need to discuss or you need to discuss with your doctor/psychiatrist whether returning to your current level or another review should occur.'

For many patients the suggestion of increasing medication or admission to hospital can increase rather than decrease their symptoms, especially where previous experiences have been unpleasant. In general, it is probably better to explore non-medical options initially and then if medication, home treatment or hospitalisation needs consideration ask the patient what they think has helped in the past. It may be possible to review this if records of use of those alternatives exist.

Obsessions

Crisis presentation of obsessional symptoms is uncommon but can give an opportunity for specific work on symptoms to begin. The symptoms may be part of a depressive or, unusually, a psychotic picture. Explanation and normalisation, where appropriate, can build on a formulation identifying key precipitants and maintaining factors. Again a rationale for intervention can help, emphasising the importance of exposure to the thoughts with response prevention (i.e. accepting the thoughts but not acting on them). Referral for longer-term cognitive behavioural work may be indicated. Use of medication would include consideration of anti-depressants, if depression is present, or anti-psychotics where psychosis is relevant. Some drugs (e.g. Clomipramine and Paroxetine) may have an effect independent of depression and although these will not have an immediate crisis relieving effect, commencement may instil hope that something can help while other measures are considered.

Feelings of unreality

Although these are not common presentations in crisis, depersonalisation and derealisation occasionally present accompanied by anxiety, depression or psychotic thoughts. Depersonalisation is a belief that you are different and have changed. The client feels distant from the world, numbed and unreal. Derealisation is where the *world* seems different: 'as if seeing it through a pane of glass'. These are thoughts related to feelings which often follow a stressful event or hallucinogenic drug experience. Normally they recede but where they persist they can become distressing and self-perpetuating. Beliefs can then arise about 'going mad' which increase anxiety and introspectiveness.

Labelling these perceptions and thoughts as depersonalisation and derealisation can in itself help as clients feel frightened, confused and isolated. Explaining that these phenomena are well recognised is always helpful. Explain their origin as being 'rather like shock': numbness can act as a protection against harsh emotion – stress – and reduce the impact of it so that the person copes with the stress gradually and calmly. Management of any underlying problems such as anxiety and depression (Chapter 5) or psychosis (see above) can reduce them, and refocusing attention on specific stresses and anxieties helps to move the client's thoughts away from the depersonalisation and derealisation.

Confusional states

Confusional states can present in community, nursing home or hospital setting (e.g. general medical wards or accident and emergency departments). Clients present with:

- altered consciousness, from over-arousal to drowsiness and coma;
- impairment of attention, registration and recall;
- disorientation in time and space, worsening during the night;
- overactivity, agitation, retardation and mutism;
- repetitive rituals;

- mood disturbance;
- thought disorder;
- delusions, especially persecutory;
- abnormal perceptions (e.g. illusions and hallucinations).

Their causes are multiple with a wide range of medical conditions able to precipitate them, such as:

- substance misuse such as drug overdose resulting in withdrawal states;
- side-effects from medication;
- infections;
- malignancies;
- endocrine disorders such as Cushing's syndrome and thyrotoxicosis;
- respiratory disorders (e.g. chronic obstructive airways disease and asthma);
- neurological conditions (e.g. brain haemorrhage – acute, sub-chronic and chronic; degenerative conditions such as dementia, multiple sclerosis and motor neurone disease);
- cardiovascular problems such as heart attacks, heart failure and congenital heart problems.

Amnesic syndrome is often associated with confusion. A client may present talking freely about past events with short-term confabulation (making up stories). Causes include Korsakov's syndrome (usually associated with alcohol dependence), encephalitis, especially viral (herpes simplex), brain trauma or post-epileptic fit.

What do you do?

Investigation and treatment of the underlying cause is obviously the way forward but in the meantime the acute disturbance needs addressing. The approach to the patient is very important. Warm, friendly conversation and clarification can reduce anxieties and agitation as rapidly as medication and has fewer side effects. This approach may need to be sustained for enduring effect (as may medication). Familiar surroundings and a reliable routine can also help. Involvement of carers can be reassuring and they can assist in passing or interpreting information about the medical condition. They can reassure the client that any management plan being established is appropriate and that the person is being looked after properly.

Taking time and considering engagement issues are worth doing even when the confusion seems profound. People who are suffering from confusion as a result of physical or psychological illness respond to clear, brief and concise communication. Medical examination should be arranged to assess physical signs of relevance.

Use of medication

Medication is usually an important component in treatment. Anti-psychotics and benzodiazepines are usually the mainstay with Haloperidol and Lorazepam frequently used. Haloperidol has the advantage over Chlorpromazine as it does not reduce blood pressure but is more likely to cause extrapyramidal side-effects. Lorazepam is short-acting and relatively safe – respiratory suppression is unusual and its short-acting nature means that if this does occur it is soon eliminated from the system while supportive measures are put in place. Its disadvantage is long-term tolerance and dependence.

A client's perspective

I found the section on delusions particularly resonant of my own experiences in crisis, and it seems well-balanced and comprehensive. What you say in the section on voices seems reasonable, and the list of coping strategies is very good. The section on medication was also very interesting, though, perhaps, there could have been more on non-pharmacological treatments.

Bob

Chapter 8

Physical symptoms

The mind-body interface still bedevils health and social care with debates continuing about who is responsible for longer-term care – whether some-body has social care or health care needs – and who should manage the crisis presentation of somebody who has social problems and physical symptoms. Within health services, debates about whether a client has a physical problem – implying the need for general medical care – or a mental health problem – correspondingly requiring mental health care, can lead to very poor services with the person and their carer being stuck in the middle and misdiagnosis and mismanagement of their problems. Crisis presentations can be passed from pillar to post, seriously increasing risk potential as a result as well as causing undue distress. Conversely, services can be dismissive or insufficiently investigate physical symptoms. Where any doubt exists, shared care and management or close liaison with a lead from one or other service are the safest routes to take. It is now more acceptable to present to health ser-vices with symptoms of 'stress', i.e. saying specifically that you are feeling depressed or anxious, but it is nevertheless also common that clients with mental health problems will present describing *physical* symptoms. This is particularly the case with older people and people from minority ethnic groups.

What are they?

Physical symptoms presenting in crisis may be due to a physical illness, or may be physical side-effects of psychiatric medication:

- tremor, stiffness, involuntary movements (jerking, twisting);
- faints, coma, urinary frequency – from diabetes or lithium toxicity;
- fever, tremor, rigidity (neuromuscular malignant syndrome);
- nausea, vomiting, headaches, dryness of mouth, constipation;
- many others . . .

They may also be the result of mental health problems:

- anxiety and depression – very varied symptoms, may be culturally determined;
- psychosis – may relate to belief system or exhaustion from overactivity;
- eating disorders – weight being a focal issue;
- substance misuse – from neglect and effects directly on the body.

Clients may present to mental health services in considerable distress with physical symptoms. Alternatively, physical symptoms and signs may emerge in discussion with them. Assessment involves understanding the relationship between the physical and psychological symptoms and the relative contribution of physical illness and mental health problems. Rarely in crisis presentations to mental health services is it one or the other, and differentiating between the contributions of each is important in management.

Presentations may involve already diagnosed physical illnesses. In these circumstances, any associated mental health problems may be:

- features of the physical illness, for example, depression with stroke or Cushing's syndrome (steroid over secretion), psychosis with HIV/AIDS, anxiety with phaeochromocytoma (tumour of adrenal glands);
- a reaction to it (e.g. depression from implication of the diagnosis, anxiety about uncertain prognosis).

As a stressor, physical illness can cause depression and dealing with it as a problem to solve or at least cope with is discussed in Chapter 5. Even where it is a feature of the illness, nonetheless medication and psychosocial interventions for the symptoms can be worth trying. Some illnesses present complex pictures and HIV/AIDS is a particular example. It can cause a wide variety of symptoms – psychosis, depression, anxiety, confusion (and cognitive deficits), delirium, anxiety and bipolar disorder. Each will need management in its own right but to complicate matters further, the anti-retroviral medication regimes used to treat AIDS can cause similar symptoms and interact with many drugs (e.g. St John's Wort, Carbamazepine and other anticonvulsants, SSRIs and benzodiazepines). Thus if any medication use is contemplated, advice from HIV specialists and pharmacists is recommended.

Presentation with physical symptoms may be because of belief that these are more likely to be taken seriously, or for cultural reasons. Presentation of depression in clients from minority ethnic groups is commonly with physical symptoms. When the assessor gives appropriate attention to mood symptoms and life circumstances, the physical symptoms may become less prominent.

Virtually any physical symptom (e.g. pain or breathlessness) and many physical signs can be a feature of anxiety ('somatisation') although there are certain distinctive signs of illness (e.g. jaundice) and investigations that can be more specific. Where a single symptom exists without other symptoms associated with anxiety, a physical cause may be more likely but nevertheless needs to be diagnosed for management to be commenced. A combination of signs and symptoms ('a syndrome') can assist in determining whether a physical illness or damage is present and also whether there are accompanying symptoms of a mental health problem, especially anxiety. However, anxiety so frequently accompanies the diagnosis and investigation of physical illness that simply determining that anxiety is present may not help in determining which condition is primary.

Where someone is suffering from mental health problems, especially where these are severe, persistent or multiple, combined with personality or learning difficulties, physical health problems are often not presented, not subject to appropriate screening or misdiagnosed. In these circumstances it becomes particularly important in crisis situations to ensure that full and sympathetic assessment occurs and, where doubt exists, that appropriate arrangements are made for continuing monitoring until that doubt is resolved.

What can you do?

Deciding whether physical symptoms require physical investigation depends on a number of factors:

- Their nature, for example:

  - severe pain;
  - sudden onset;
  - position of pain (e.g. chest, head or lower abdomen);
  - change in consciousness level;
  - rapid fluctuations in mood state;
  - hallucinations, especially visual or olfactory (of smell).

- Physical signs:

  - pallor or cyanosis (blueness of skin);
  - shortness of breath;
  - pain on examination;
  - confusion in time and space.

- Occurrence:

  - first episode;
  - similarity to symptom (e.g. pain, or sign previously diagnosed as physical disease).

Certain physical conditions are particularly recognised as producing symptoms similar to anxiety:

- phaeochromocytoma (tumour of adrenal glands);
- thyrotoxicosis (overactive thyroid);
- cardiac disease (e.g. supra-ventricular tachycardia, causing rapid heart beat experienced as palpitations);
- hypoglycaemia (low blood sugar);
- medication side-effects.

Physical symptoms require physical investigation unless there is very good reason not to do so. A medically or nursing trained mental health practitioner may be able to reach an appropriate conclusion about the symptoms themselves. Others may wish to seek an opinion from a medical team member, nurse triage system (e.g. NHS Direct in the UK), hospital or family doctor. The degree of urgency is determined by the apparent severity or nature of the symptoms.

Accompanying the person to the medical examination or deciding whether an ambulance needs to be called depends on the apparent urgency of the situation and, in the former instance, your availability. However, if the latter is an issue, arrangements to obtain the services of a carer, advocate, support worker or other mental health practitioner need to be considered.

As mentioned previously, people with mental health problems are more likely to develop physical illnesses. The complication is that anxiety, depression, schizophrenia and other disorders may present with physical symptoms which can be difficult to differentiate. It is better to be safe and apparently waste time on a medical assessment and intervention than miss treatable physical illness – or even untreatable but diagnosable illness. This is because it allows the client to decide how to deal with it. It also is because treatment of non-existent mental health problems is pointless and potentially can lead to such problems (e.g. anxiety), and any coexisting mental health problems can also be tricky to treat with significant doubt remaining.

After a medical examination or where it is concluded that such an examination is not appropriate (e.g. where the description of the pattern of symptoms has not changed since previous investigation), the distress the person is experiencing will need a response.

Always remember that the apparent absence of a physical diagnosis does not mean no illness exists. A continued level of scepticism is appropriate and can be communicated to the patient: 'Although no physical illness has been found, we will remain alert to any possibility that one exists. However, it may still be worth seeing if there are other ways of helping you with how you feel.'

Depending on the symptom, explaining how stress (probably a better, more acceptable term than anxiety or depression) can cause 'real' physical symptoms may be helpful. Discussing 'cramp' resulting from muscle overuse – but not disease – can be useful. Explanation that when stressed and tense this can happen all over the body can reduce anxiety. Effects of hyperventilation can be discussed and even produced to illustrate symptoms such as breathlessness etc. Leaflets can be useful to back this up and examples from these described. The basic assumption that needs discussion is that a physical symptom can only be produced by physical disease. Assessment may have identified reasons why the person is particularly likely to identify physical symptoms as problematic. For example, the person has:

- a relative who has recently died or become ill;
- become ill themselves, and this is particularly an issue for them;
- been misdiagnosed;
- found the condition to be particularly distressing;
- a dependent or antagonistic relationship with another;
- been or feels blamed for an event.

Disentangling these issues can be effective even in the crisis situation. Establishing why and how appropriate guilt or blame is apportioned and collaborating over a balanced and accurate assessment can clarify and refocus concerns. Ask the client:

- What did you do?
- Why was that wrong?
- What could you reasonably have done?

Misdiagnosis may require a plan of action. It may be appropriate to review whether the misdiagnosis was such that seeking further explanation by the diagnostician is reasonable (e.g. through direct approach or complaints procedures). Establishing what to do or what not to do can in itself reduce distress.

Crises can result from distress around the presence of and response to significant illness, which may be newly diagnosed. Most people reach for the support of friends or family, or possibly the person supplying them with the information. Discussion with the client should address:

- current issues (e.g. pain or disability);
- future fears (e.g. of overwhelming pain or death);
- a problem-solving approach;
- effectiveness of any prescribed pain relief.

It is not possible to give an absolute guarantee of pain relief but explanation of the availability of strong painkillers and of their relative effectiveness is helpful. Individuals will want to strike a balance between the effectiveness of pain relief, adverse effects and the effects on their functioning. Many people want to remain reasonably alert, which may mean tolerating some pain, provided the option of increased pain relief exists. They may also wish to keep active, even if that means pain (e.g. from an arthritic hip). Explicitly setting out these options and enabling the person to make choices can defuse crises.

The client may fear the prospect of dying and sensitively exploring this can be helpful where it seems to be a key issue. Often it emerges that other issues are key, such as fear of:

- pain;
- disfigurement;
- leaving others unsupported;
- dying alone;
- the unknown.

These can each be explored and allayed, solutions planned and situations prepared for. Evaluating what can be done and accepting what cannot can relieve anxiety. Religious belief can be worth exploring in these circumstances in the broadest sense and support from spiritual advisers enlisted.

Depression and anxiety symptoms are discussed in Chapter 5 and advice on management will be of relevance if the client accepts that mental health issues are relevant. Even where they don't, they may independently accept support in managing their problems and this can subsequently have a beneficial effect on their symptoms.

Eating disorders

Eating disorders include bulimia and anorexia nervosa. Obesity is not considered here as it does not yet present as a sole issue in mental health crises, although it can certainly contribute to them. Weight gain can affect self-esteem and result in anxiety and depression and can also be a significant side-effect of anti-psychotic medication.

Bulimia

Presentation of bulimia nervosa in crisis is unusual but generally involves issues to do with self-harm, substance misuse, depression and anxiety. However, physical complications such as blood test abnormalities (electrolytes) related to use of laxatives can occur. If the latter present, it will usually be through the client's family doctor who has found these abnormalities after routine investigation or following through physical symptoms presenting to them.

What can you do?

Where associated symptoms present, ways of working in crisis will use the principles outlined in the relevant chapters. However, it may still be possible and necessary to provide assistance for the bulimic issues themselves. This

---

Box 8.1 Bulimia and anorexia

Bulimia nervosa

Features include:

- recurrent binge eating;
- sense of lack of control over eating;
- self-induced vomiting;
- laxative, diuretic or enema misuse;
- fasting;
- excessive exercise;
- may have normal or high body weight;
- focus on body shape and image;
- distress, impulsivity and self-harm.

Anorexia

Features include:

- low body weight (<85% of expected);
- intense fear of gaining weight or becoming fat;
- absence of periods (amenorrhoea);
- binge eating and vomiting;
- excessive exercise;
- laxative, diuretic and enema misuse;
- distress, impulsivity and self-harm.

---

can be done directly by introducing some of the principles of effective treatment of bulimia at a stage when motivation to make changes is relatively good. Or it may be that the person is presenting at a time when they are receiving treatment already but going through a difficult period. Keeping to the treatment programme may be proving difficult, they may be getting demoralised and they may have relapsed into bingeing. Understanding the principles of therapy can be useful to them and their therapist in helping them get back on track. The evidence for the effectiveness of cognitive behavioural and interpersonal therapies is good and explaining this can help with motivation and instil hope for the future.

Work will always involve an individualised formulation to identify issues that need to be dealt with in their own right. Managing diet and exercise will be important using food and mood diary-keeping, having a regular meal pattern and combating the common belief that 'if I eat normally, I'll gain weight'. Self-help manuals[1] can help with this where bulimia is relatively uncomplicated or while awaiting therapy.

Anti-depressants have a limited role, being effective in an estimated 25 per cent of cases, but this is frequently not maintained in the longer-term. Higher doses (e.g. Fluoxetine, 60mg daily), are used and use is not dependent on having comorbid depression. Clients generally will not take those anti-depressants which include weight gain as a side-effect.

Anorexia

Weight loss can present for psychological or physical reasons in crisis, usually as a symptom associated with depression and anxiety but also with psychosis associated with voices commanding the client not to eat or beliefs that their food is being poisoned. Self-harm and substance misuse may also feature. Sometimes carers will present the client to services with concerns that they are losing weight, even though the client sees nothing wrong with this. Indeed they may believe that they are fat – they have a 'distorted body image'.

What can you do?

Where perception of body image is not disturbed, management will generally be directed towards individual presenting features (e.g. depression, self-harm or psychosis). Possible physical causes always need to be considered and investigated.

It is clearly important to determine the degree of weight loss and length of time over which it has been occurring. Where the weight loss is not an immediate cause for concern (i.e. the vast majority of instances) in crisis it may well be better to concentrate on understanding the concerns of the carers and client and try to broaden the discussion away from weight and diet. Working with the person's strengths as part of managing the crisis can assist – for example, what do they have in their lives apart from the eating disorder? When clients are already known to services some crisis planning may have been done and can be drawn on if available. If part of the prevention has been, for example, to get the person into college, discussion can be about that and how it can help with friendships and boosting self-esteem. This approach moves the focus away from a battle over food. Reassessment after the immediate crisis is over can then occur and appropriate support be arranged. The carers may need to know that immediate risk to health is not an issue while agreeing with them that help is needed and will be offered.

Clients with a longer-term history of anorexia, usually but not always already known to services, can occasionally and potentially disastrously present in crisis to non-specialist teams. Assessment of risk can be fraught, with limited cooperation from the client combined with complicated carer responses. Suicidality may be a significant risk and there are also risks to physical health from the consequences of low body weight and electrolyte imbalance (e.g. from the use of laxatives). While involvement of specialist services in making immediate assessment is usually desirable, it is not always available. However, discussion with them may still be possible and valuable. Assessment of weight reduction always needs to include consideration of physical causes (e.g. a physical illness such as diabetes or malignancy), and consequences. Generally this is better done by the person's family doctor who has the relevant medical records and expertise which may necessitate conveying the person to such an appointment urgently. Where nurse screening services are available this may be a route for rapid access to services or if not, the use of an accident and emergency department. Further investigation may be necessary by specialist services. A medically trained member of the mental health team may also be able to perform this initial screening, dependent on their recent training and expertise. Liaison with the family doctor will always be vital with these patients.

Principles of risk assessment and management in this context are similar to those generally used (see Chapter 2) but with the special complication of weight loss. Weighing is essential where serious danger to health is posed. Estimating the body mass index (BMI) (weight (kg)/height (cm)^2) is very valuable, but a safe BMI is very individual. Nevertheless if a patient has a BMI under 15 or has had a very rapid reduction in weight, specialist advice should be taken – either from the local eating disorders service, or via contact with the nearest regional services or national centres.

Cooperation can be a major issue (e.g. with weighing). A collaborative approach is the most effective in the longer term but sometimes the persuasion needed has to utilise every possible argument available and involve family, and even discussion of which scales can be used. Estimation of weight is difficult without weighing and patients are adept at concealing their weight. Appearance can assist where weighing is refused if the person is looking emaciated, but exact weight is essential to determine whether compulsory measures are necessary. If not emaciated, there may be time – days or weeks – to negotiate over weighing.

Management of the crisis may involve reinstituting a treatment and eating regime. Strict behavioural programmes are less favoured now but more informal 'reward' systems can have their place even if this just involves taking time to explain the benefits of eating just that little bit more and the inevitable consequences of not doing so. Where activity is excessive, reduction in it may help but decisions over confinement to bed are probably better developed as part of a longer-term regime, if used at all.

Discussion of the use of laxatives is necessary. Explain how useless they are in weight loss. Diuretics can also be misused and although when commenced the may have a marginal impact, this is lost immediately afterwards.

The next stage can involve home treatment or, less desirable, admission to hospital and worse still, regimes involving refeeding (including by tube).

Developing a 'threatening' position is very easy to do but can polarise discussion with family and client. Using an explanatory collaborative approach is usually more successful. However, the evidence base for intervention is poor, even for cognitive behavioural approaches which might have been thought to be effective, and there is no substitute currently for getting advice from experienced specialist practitioners.

Mental health legislation would normally only be invoked when weight loss is life threatening. However, detention in hospital can lead to increasingly dysfunctional behaviour and be counterproductive in the longer term. Again advice from eating disorder specialists is valuable – if only by providing support for difficult decisions. Liaison between all parties can ensure that communication to family and the client is consistent and that risk issues are fully and continually assessed and management jointly agreed.

Family work has a long-term place but short-term collaboration is also valuable. The family often present 'at their wits end', so calmly taking control of the situation, having collaboratively assessed it, and repudiating any suggestions that they might be to blame may help. Crises can be protracted and require management over days or weeks in which a process of negotiation and goal-setting is tried and retried. Even though past behaviour suggests that compulsory measures are going to be inevitable, the negotiation process may help with longer-term management.

Case example

Jane, aged 22, was presented by her family urgently because of concerns that she was 'wasting away'. She had come very reluctantly and initially refused to speak. She was asked if she wanted to be seen on her own and did request this. She then said that her ex-boyfriend had always called her fat. Following their break-up she had returned to live with her parents. She was feeling low but denied being depressed. She agreed to being weighed and her BMI was calculated at 16.

Jane's parent's were invited back in, with her agreement, and were reassured that her current weight was safe. However, their concerns about Jane's loss of weight, estimated at two stone in three months, were such that the mental health practitioner agreed to contact the local eating disorder service (EDS) and ask if they would consider assessing the family. In the meantime arrangements were made for Jane to have an anti-depressant – Fluoxetine – although she was unsure about taking it. A contact number was given and a promise made to telephone them following the discussion with the EDS.

Bizarre physical symptoms

Bizarre physical symptoms sometimes present which do not appear to fit any diagnostic category or appear delusional in content (e.g. 'my brain has been

---

Box 8.2 Eating disorders checklist

Bulimia:

- Focus on work with individual behaviours and any mood problems.
- Use opportunity to explain basic cognitive behaviour therapy and consider referral.

Anorexia:

- Try to develop engagement before addressing weight issues.
- Assess (including observation of build) if the situation now becoming dangerous: if not, negotiate and try to engage in a longer-term therapeutic approach or refer to EDS; if so, weigh and estimate BMI.
- If client refuses to be weighed or BMI <15 or rapidly dropping toward that, contact EDS to discuss. If there is no local EDS, consider ringing national or regional services. Consider on basis of degree of emaciation and advice from specialist services whether to resort to compulsory admission.

---

removed by aliens' or 'my body is rotting away' or 'my body is infested'). It is reasonable to have a high index of suspicion that symptoms that 'don't fit' may have a physical cause and not dismiss them as psychological in origin, especially where other psychological symptoms are not present or explainable by quite reasonable anxiety. This may mean considering more extensive investigation and consultation with medical colleagues.

The symptoms may be an inarticulate or unusual attempt to describe something that the person finds indescribable or may be part of a psychotic syndrome. Where mood is very depressed, Cotard's syndrome has been described, where the belief exists that part of the body is diseased or rotting or death is imminent or has even occurred. In these circumstances, treatment of depression is appropriate with use of anti-psychotics or electroconvulsive therapy. Where depression does not appear to be the major cause, symptoms can be single – a monosymptomatic hypochondriacal delusional psychosis or part of a broader picture with other psychotic symptoms as part of schizophrenia. Treatment of the psychosis is appropriate using anti-psychotics, psychological and social interventions (see Chapter 7).

Stupor

Stupor, or unresponsiveness, while appearing conscious, is a very uncommon presentation but may present in hospital settings. Causes include: depression, dementia, schizophrenia, akinetic mutism – with disturbance in level of consciousness, ictal (epileptic fit) and post-ictal states, encephalitis or encephalopathies, damage to frontal or temporal brain lobes or posterior diencephalon, Parkinson's disease, anti-psychotic overdose, hypo- or hyperglycaemia, or uraemia. It is generally safest to assume stupor to be organic in cause until shown to be otherwise. Management involves investigation of possible causes and then observation. Where psychological phenomena are the cause, the client will usually emerge from the stupor. Gentle conversation and explanation, especially if the client needs any investigations or procedures, or, as they emerge, help with eating and drinking, can develop a relationship and reduce fear and anxiety, encouraging communication.

Physically ill and refusing treatment

Advice is sometimes asked in crisis where a person with a diagnosed physical illness is requiring treatment but refusing it. In these circumstances their competence to make decisions becomes relevant (see Chapter 3).

What can you do?

If they are competent, it may be appropriate to:

- discuss alternative treatment plans that may be more acceptable to the client even if not medically ideal;
- address any grievances that the client has about their treatment so far – or the treatment of others, such as friends and relatives, which is now affecting their decision;
- assess and try to allay any fears that exist (e.g. needle or operation phobia);
- ensure that full information in a form that can be understood has been given and any false or incomplete information corrected;
- involve any carer – informal or formal – or friend who is prepared to assist.

If they continue to refuse any treatment, it is important to document this and it may be reasonable to return to the discussion later.

If a decision is made that the client is lacking competence, it is possible to act in their best interests, taking into account any wishes they may have expressed in advance of the decision (e.g. through an advance directive). If their decision-making is impaired by a mental disorder, consider whether the use of mental health legislation is appropriate to enforce treatment of a medical or surgical problem. If the mental disorder is not related to the physical problem, such enforcement of treatment would not be appropriate. However, if competence to make the decision is compromised by the understanding of the physical illness and/or management and the implications of not accepting treatment, through mental disorder, it is possible to treat. In these circumstances, in practice most physicians and surgeons will wish to obtain supporting legal advice.

No physical illness or mental health problems found

Presentation with physical symptoms where no physical illness or mental health problems are found can occur in relation to:

- concern that they may be ill: reassurance that they are not can lead to the crisis being over;
- substance misuse, especially where the person is trying to get opiates;
- desire for accommodation;
- desire to avoid legal difficulties;
- desire for a caring response from others (although whether this is ever deliberate is difficult to demonstrate); this may relate to past psychological difficulties or previous treatment in hospital.

So-called 'Munchausen's syndrome' is presentation of factitious physical symptoms which may be related to past relationship problems (personality disorder). Presentation tends to be with abdominal pain, haematuria (blood in urine), pyrexia (fever) of unknown origin, rashes and chest pain. There may be:

- unwillingness to give personal details;
- claims to be away from home;
- elaborate but implausible explanations (pseudologia fantastica);
- classical symptom presentation which seems 'too good to be true' (perhaps reflecting rehearsal of presentation or repeats of it);
- family or personal links with medical or nursing profession, or lengthy hospital stays early in life;
- history of substance misuse.

Psychological Munchausen's has also been described where clients imitate psychotic presentations. Munchausen's by proxy is the highly controversial syndrome where the client's children or elderly dependents are presented with induced or falsely described physical symptoms.

What can you do?

Diagnosing factitious symptoms can be very difficult and unless there is clear evidence of deceit, it is usually safer to investigate and treat on the basis of what is presented because:

- what seems factitious may not be – it may be a problem with communication or cultural interpretation;
- where the person has previously presented with factitious symptoms, they can still develop physical illness and mental health problems and are probably more likely to do so than the general population.

While it may reinforce the pattern of presentations to treat, it is still the safest option unless there is clear evidence of previous similar presentations. It is always important to reassess in case a change has occurred. Offering psychological support needs consideration – for substance misuse, if that is the issue, or for general assessment if matters are more complex. Issues which may be treatable, such as depression, PTSD or borderline personality disorder may emerge.

A client's perspective

This is pretty much as I have experienced it in practice and as a carer.

Carmel

Chapter 9

Service teams and settings

There are a plethora of teams that make up specialist mental health services. Clients, carers and new staff members can be forgiven for finding it a bewildering process to work out what services they should be using, liaising with or referring to. As well as the inpatient and the generic community teams providing services there are usually a number of specialist teams. Some will be within the main community team and some run separately, depending on the policy of the particular mental health service. The teams that may potentially exist in one area are shown in Figure 9.1.

Services for children, adolescents and older people will also exist but these

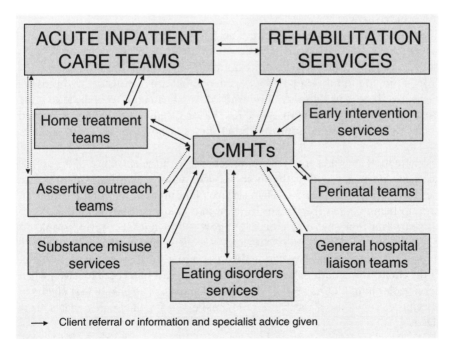

→ Client referral or information and specialist advice given

Figure 9.1 Service provision

tend to be more straightforward with specific community teams for these groups. However, early intervention services are increasingly seeing younger clients (sometimes down to age 14). Problems with referrals and interfaces with these services are unlikely to arise in crisis situations and so they are not discussed further.

Clients generally should not be transferred when in a crisis so contact in these situations is likely to be for advice from colleagues who have a particular specialist expertise. There may be issues in a crisis about inpatient beds, for example if an adult client has pre-senile dementia, an older person's inpatient care may be more appropriate. Adolescent services will sometimes want to place young people in adult wards because of their physical size and behaviour. The balance to be struck is between consideration that these environments are rarely the right placement for distressed and vulnerable teenagers against the undesirability of sending them a long way away from family and friends.

Forensic services tend to manage their clients' crises within forensic settings and immediate crisis assessments in the community are usually not available, although at a later time they may become so, once the initial situation is stabilised in hospital or the community (sometimes involving holding in police custody). There are often staff in generic services with some forensic experience that may be able to provide advice, such as those who see clients through the court system before they reach forensic services and those running low secure services.

Statutory teams outside mental health services altogether need to be remembered. In crisis work there will often be a need to co-work with colleagues from other services, for example, the learning disability services or from child and family teams. In assessments that are to consider compulsory measures there is usually a rota of available qualified staff to undertake these on a geographical basis. In the UK, this is often organised by approved social workers or other approved practitioners who cover all client services and ages.

There are key issues for crisis management with the existence of a number of specialist teams within the main service, mainly regarding the interface between the different teams. When service planning is at its worst, clients can end up being passed from team to team in a crisis, perhaps being 'assessed' three or four times before a plan of support is drawn up. However, people do not come in one-dimensional 'packages' – a client may need an alternative to admission, but also have an eating disorder and a substance misuse problem. If the client is pregnant as well the whole system can snarl up. However, when service planning is at its best, having specialist teams can ensure that clients in specific circumstances receive a tailor-made service that really meets their needs.

We will begin by giving a description of all the teams that clients may come across to assist with considering whether seeking advice or referral is appropriate in a specific crisis. We will spend some time in examining the roles and responsibilities of each, particularly in relation to crisis presentations and how they may present differently to individual teams. We will finally make some suggestions as to how the interface between teams can be negotiated to provide the best service with the least duplication.

Community mental health teams

What are they?

These are the locality teams, sometimes known as care management teams, that have taken responsibility for the care of clients in the community since the closure or restructuring of hospital-based services. Social policy in most countries has been to reduce long-stay inpatient care and move services to the community. This has also been a response to clients' general preferences to receive services in their own home or locality. Teams are based on population groups, usually defined geographically, sometimes by specific contract (e.g. with a state or insurance organisation), or by family medical practices (as often occurs in the UK).

A CMHT[1] will be staffed by a number of professionals from different disciplines who will bring their particular expertise to the team. In a typical team there are likely to be mental health nurses, social workers, psychiatrists, occupational therapists, psychologists, administration staff and support workers. Within this group of staff, there may well be individuals who take a particular role, for example in group work or in working with clients who are involved in the criminal justice system, and others who manage the interface with forensic services. Clients are often seen in their own homes and practitioners work with clients to produce support packages that promote recovery and maximise quality of life.

A community team manager or individuals within the team will also often hold a budget for the purchase of care for clients in that area (e.g. for domiciliary care packages, residential care or sometimes transport costs for clients to access services). As with health and social care everywhere, resources are limited and priorities have to be set.

What do they do?

Most teams work with those people who have severe and enduring mental health problems. They are also likely to pick up people who are being discharged from inpatient care. Some teams are in a position to do more work that is preventative in nature, by running clinics in primary care settings or by short-term work with people who are becoming unwell. Whatever the size and breadth of the individual team, it is certainly from this sort of team that the majority of clients will receive their mental health care. It is usually to these teams that a GP will initially refer a client with problems and it is often the decision of such teams to refer the client on to specialist teams that exist in the locality. Teams are likely to offer the following:

*   assessment of new referrals of people with potential mental health diffi-culties – urgent, immediate or routine;
*   short- and long-term psychosocial interventions by care coordinators for those with severe and/or enduring mental health problems;
*   some group work around particular issues (e.g. abuse or hearing voices) or around skills (e.g. assertiveness or anxiety management).
*   gatekeeping for services such as day services or care management;
*   some therapies: psychological and maybe complementary;
*   psychiatric outpatient and domiciliary services and medication manage-ment;
*   depot medication administration;
*   support of carers;
*   support in accessing occupation and leisure activities;
*   the provision of a duty service.

The whole range of crises described in this book can present to these teams, requiring assessment and management as discussed.

How crises are managed

Crises in CMHTs tend to be dealt with by a duty service or worker unless the client is already known and allocated to a worker within the team who happens to be available. The duty service means a practitioner (or a number of practitioners) who has put time aside from their usual work just to deal with any new referrals, general enquiries, requests for advice or indeed any crisis presentations that may come up. The staff that cover this service are likely to be qualified and are (usually) non-medical staff. There is then usually a parallel system of medical duty cover, although increasingly these are being integrated in a multi-disciplinary way. As most crisis presentations come to the CMHT, it is at this point that the decision gets made about who is to respond to the situation and undertake the necessary assessment. We will discuss some guidelines for deciding who should provide the initial assessment later in this chapter, but the important role for the CMHT duty worker is the 'triage' role, the gathering of the initial information, often over the telephone, which will inform the final decision.

Inpatient teams

Inpatient care remains an integral and indispensable part of all mental health systems, but its role has been changing rapidly. Admission criteria vary considerably, particularly where effective teams are operating (e.g. CMHTs, assertive outreach or especially home treatment) and where effective bed management strategies are in place. There is a full discussion of who should be admitted to inpatient settings in Chapter 4. Unnecessary hospitalisation is damaging to the individual's coping abilities and often their self-esteem.

What are they?

Inpatient teams work with clients who are admitted to hospital for their mental health care. They include nurses, psychiatrists and unqualified support workers in the main but most wards should have occupational therapy and pharmacy input and some have access to psychological services. A range of inpatient settings exist. The most common are acute admission units and rehabilitation units but there are also low-secure or intensive care wards and medium- and high-secure wards. There are also a small number of specialist units for eating disorders and psychosis. There will be some differences in the type of crises presenting in these different settings, with risk issues being more prominent and complex in the higher secure environments, however the underlying issues giving rise to crises are likely to be similar in each environment. In rehabilitation settings, similarities to acute inpatient settings will be greater the higher the level of nursing staff available, especially if they are sited on hospital premises. As the levels of support reduce, so the similarities lessen and crisis presentations become essentially crises in the community.

Most clients use acute inpatient services because they are in a crisis and cannot be adequately supported at home. The very process of going into hospital can be traumatic, particularly if the admission is not voluntary. Inpatients are out of their own environment, although they may still maintain contact with it through leave arrangements, and the staff are working with a lot of people who are unsettled and out of equilibrium.

Given the importance of this work with the most vulnerable and distressed clients, it is very sad that the status of inpatient units in mental health services has become so low. The retention of nursing staff on the wards has been a difficulty in many areas. The growth of specialist teams has taken many of the most experienced nursing staff away from the wards, although there is a shortage of nursing staff in general. Whatever the reasons, wards in some areas have to depend on staff from recruitment agencies that may not know the clients and are unable to offer continuity of care at a time when it is most needed. Various initiatives are attempting to address this.[2]

Service users report serious concerns about inpatient units[3] regarding:

- poor physical and psychological environment for care, including lack of basic necessities and arrangements for safety, privacy, dignity and comfort;

- insufficient information on clients' condition and treatment and on how the ward and service operates;
- lack of involvement and engagement in the planning and review of care and in how the ward is run;
- inadequate staff contact, particularly one-to-one contact;
- insufficient attention to the importance of such key factors as ethnicity and gender, and protection from harassment/abuse;
- lack of 'something to do', especially activity that is useful and meaningful to recovery.

The environment provided by some units has improved and is now very good – clean, tidy and homely – but in many it is still appalling and this is certainly a factor in aggravating and even precipitating crises. Distress will be increased in poor surroundings; behaviour can worsen and nursing care can be that much more difficult. Not surprisingly, clients will also be reluctant to be admitted, leading to unnecessary use of compulsory measures at times.

Once someone is admitted to inpatient care, it is easy to fall into the trap, for community staff, of believing that crisis management or prevention is over. However, anyone who has worked in such settings will be aware that this is certainly not the case. The circumstances of acute wards and the nature of the problems that people are admitted with mean that crises are ever present. Many clients do not want to be there – and are only there because there is nowhere more suitable for them to go because of accommodation shortages or because they are detained under mental health legislation. Resurgence of psychotic symptoms or suicidality, panic or behavioural disorder occurs on a day-to-day basis and management of these crises is necessary.

What do they do?

The bulk of work on wards is about supporting clients to manage crises and preparing them for living elsewhere. For some clients there is also a need to protect them from risk to self or others. A new admission is likely to be a person in crisis and that person is likely to have had at least one assessment if not several in the 24 hours or so before admission. The initial work on the ward involves engagement with them, introduction to the new environment for the client, collecting vital information and establishing the level of support and observation that will be needed. An assessment and nursing care plan will be established and then built up with the client over time and after discussion in nurse meetings and multidisciplinary ward reviews. There can be advantages to being in a new place and away from the sources of distress. Some clients talk of the help they got from having the 'time out' that came from being in hospital, to be able to adjust while being away from the pressures of everyday life.

The decision about the level of observation of the client required will be a joint one between nursing staff and the admitting doctor. This should not be affected by staff levels available, but where staffing is too low to provide the levels determined it is important to involve more senior doctors and nurse managers to safely resolve the situation. Their reassessment of risk may lead to a decision that high levels of observation are not required, or that other staff can be drafted in from elsewhere, or that the client needs to be nursed in a safer environment (e.g. a psychiatric intensive care or low-secure unit). Levels of care are described as:[4]

- *general*: location of client known to staff at all times, contact with staff at each shift;
- *intermittent*: location checked every 15–30 minutes, exact time specified;
- *within eyesight*: day or night;
- *within arms length*: more than one member of staff may be needed.

Many of the principles and practice described elsewhere for management of mental health problems are applicable in inpatient units although their circumstances and lack of staff can mean that taking time out to work through a crisis with someone can be very difficult. Sometimes this means that though the crisis may continue for the individual, it has to wait until time becomes available for it to be worked with. It may be that partial and sequential working through occurs as and when the staff member can assist – having a good memory and a structured and evolving crisis management plan can make a huge difference in cases like this.

There are a number of key problems for managing crises in an inpatient setting which are about the setting itself.

- People associate hospitals with medical symptoms and approaches.

  o The focus on managing the crisis in such a setting can be biological and centred on medication. This can be reinforced by psychiatric and nursing attitudes but the mere fact of being in hospital may invite the client to see their distress in medical terms. They may not see the relevance of the precipitating factors that led up to the episode unless they are specifically invited to.
  o The social and psychological circumstances involved in hospitalisation will inevitably need to be addressed if discharge is to occur and readmission avoided.

- The person in hospital may behave in an institutional way.

  o This can be like a person in hospital is 'meant' to behave – as a patient, a recipient of care. This can lead to a passivity that staff end up getting frustrated about.
  o There are also other institutional behaviours that can impede

recovery, such as clients feeling rebellious against a (seemingly) authoritarian regime and becoming verbally aggressive or persistently rule-breaking. This is more likely to be the case if staff take a 'parent' voice to clients who are inpatients. Some of the principles used in transactional analysis[5] can be helpful in keeping 'adult to adult' interactions going rather than the 'parent–child' roles that develop so easily.

- The client is often disempowered by the hospital setting and collaboration in care planning can be problematic.

   ○ This can be due to the dominance of the 'ward round' in the planning of care. These are often large meetings involving doctors, nurses, students, therapists and pharmacists, and hidden somewhere within is the voice of the client. Attending a large meeting of powerful professionals is stressful for somebody in good health and it is expecting rather a lot to ask clients to feel confident to express any, let alone a contrary, opinion in such a setting. Many nurses try to counter this by helping clients write down their views beforehand and by the use of advocates in ward reviews. It is also important to allow the client time in a smaller gathering (e.g. psychiatrist and key nurse), to discuss important issues, if they wish to, even though this can be disruptive to the 'ward round' process.

   ○ Involvement of community agencies in discharge planning, the requirements of training and multidisciplinary review, can lead to large meetings but the needs and wishes of the individual client need to have priority.

Questions often arise about whether to continue or discontinue admission: 'I want to leave now'. Decisions are determined particularly in relation to risk issues. Such consideration has to be long- and short-term. For example, continuing an admission when substances have been misused contrary to contract/agreement, or behaviour has been verbally or physically aggressive or simply obstructive, may seem safer in the short-term for the individual. But protecting the person from the consequences of their behaviour can lead to it continuing and make the inevitable rejection by services, and society more generally, more devastating and dangerous. The potential damage to others within the ward, both patients and staff, has also to be weighed up. Continuing support is usually appropriate to offer where inpatient admission has been deemed appropriate initially. Sometimes where admission has occurred unplanned and out of hours and no continuing mental health support will help, this may not be appropriate.

What happens post-admission when the client gets passed back to community services depends on a range of factors. Most clients will get passed back to the CMHT as the recognised hub of the outpatient service. This may be for short-term follow up, day care, outpatient care or for more long-term support or therapy. The client may be referred to a specialist team directly if they are assessed as having a very specific problem (e.g. an eating disorder or a need for rehabilitation services). They may have been involved with those teams prior to admission and be well supported there. Hospital discharge does not necessarily mean crisis resolution has occurred and indeed many clients are returning to the same social stresses they had prior to admission. Suicide rates increase in the week after discharge and remain elevated over the next year, so follow-up is therefore vital in crisis prevention.

Hospital is the one setting where response to aggressive behaviour (see Chapter 6) can involve seclusion or restraint, but these responses need to be in accordance with an agreed policy, proportional to the risks involved, necessary (the principle of necessity under English common law applies) and documented appropriately. Training in management of aggressive behaviour and specifically control and restraint is a necessary precursor to involvement in situations where it may be used. Prevention of the escalation of circumstances leading to restraint and seclusion is the ultimate goal, and having sufficient trained staff to enable this to happen is clearly a benefit to all concerned.

Attention also needs to be paid to the interpersonal consequences of client behaviour on the ward. A code of conduct should identify clearly unacceptable behaviour such as racial or sexual harassment, or theft. This should also cover ward rules, negotiated with service users, regarding housekeeping issues such as management of noise (TVs, radios, etc.) and how disputes – often crises – over such matters are to be resolved.

Reasons for admission include:

- Significant risk of serious harm to self or others (see Chapter 6).

  - Expressed suicidal intent.
  - Expressed homicidal intent or serious threat of physical harm to others.
  - Suicidal planning or serious harm to others with uncertainty about intent.
  - Suicidal thinking where there is concern that this might abruptly change to intent (e.g. where there is foreknowledge of catastrophic news affecting the person or past history of this occurring).
  - Command hallucinations with demonstrated 'control override', i.e. the person believes they have to act in accordance with the commands of the voice(s) and does something to make this apparent.
  - Severe physical neglect (e.g. caused by anorexia nervosa, mania or when client presents late with depression or psychosis).

- As an alternative to living at home or where homeless.

  - Home treatment is not possible without a home; however admission to hospital cannot be the most appropriate option in these circumstances although its convenience is such that it is frequently used. Better alternatives are to use local homelessness provision and liaison with local housing department. Discussions about temporary options (e.g. friends and family) may be possible.

○ Few services have respite options available (e.g. supported flats or crisis accommodation). It is more sensible, economic and less damaging to fund guesthouse accommodation, 'foster' homes, crisis houses or crisis beds in hostel accommodation.

- Intensive or specialised care is required.

○ Commencement on the anti-psychotic Clozapine may be safer to do in hospital because of potential adverse reactions, but partial hospitalisation or community options, especially with home treatment support, may be better.

○ ECT, where there is concern about physical status, although day patient options can be explored.

- Patient preference for hospital admission.

○ Previous positive experience.
○ Feeling need for the perceived safety of admission.
○ 'Unable to cope' with demands of home life.
○ Escape from home circumstances where they may feel at risk or under pressure from family (including domestic violence).

- Carers are no longer able to cope.

○ Alternatives not available or acceptable to client or carer (although this may not seem a sufficient reason, at times not agreeing can lead to a greater crisis, increased risk or the carer not being prepared to continue in that role).

- Combined risk, preference and other considerations such as presence or absence of assertive outreach or home treatment service may make admission inevitable and appropriate.

Day service teams

Day hospitals and day care are available in most areas but have varied functions and often quite confused roles. Rather like inpatient units, as new teams have emerged, they have often become depleted of staff and attention.

The term day hospital tends to be used to mean a place where the focus is on people who have relatively acute symptoms and who attend for a relatively brief period of time. Generally this means no more than three to six months although frequently exceptions are made. Sometimes they are in the same building as inpatient wards or alongside a community mental health centre, or may be separately located in a community setting. Group and individual activities are provided for the purposes of anxiety management, assertiveness, art or occupational therapy, recreation and social skills, with the objective of providing an alternative to admission to hospital. It has been demonstrated that day hospitals can be effective in doing this. They may also provide intensive input to manage depressive symptoms and support the provision of outpatient ECT.

Day care tends to mean services provided in day centres or clubs, often run by social service departments or non-statutory organisations, which provide a range of social, creative, occupational and other therapeutic activities. Some will run groups on symptom management or relaxation and have services for particular groups of clients (e.g. women, men, black people or younger people). There may be assistance with vocational advice and associated skills. Clients attend for as long as their mental health problems warrant it and many day centres can become a long-term lifeline for service users. They meet a need for company and meaningful occupation and some are open at weekends or evenings when clients may need support.

What can they do?

Day services provide support for people who have presented in crisis and clients and staff may encounter and manage such crises in these settings. In fact, some clients attend day services several times a week and it is therefore to the day services that a client may turn if they are experiencing difficulties, and their advice to other teams about the client's problems can be valuable. Clients may develop roles within day centres, such as providing peer support, running user-led groups or advocacy.

Day services can frequently manage crises themselves but may ask for help from the client's care coordinators in other teams. The principles and practice described elsewhere apply here. Managing and having the confidence to manage crises effectively can mean that maintaining support for individuals after the crisis occurs is possible. Unfortunately crises can lead to exclusion from facilities and while disruption to activities and others' equilibrium needs to be considered, if day care and day hospitals are to be most valuable for those who can most benefit from them, coping effectively with crises and minimising turbulence are necessary skills for staff to develop with the appropriate support and training. Often explanations to other group members in general or specific terms, where clients give permission, can allay their anxieties and enlist their support to help the client avoid or cope better with future crises.

Home treatment/crisis resolution teams

Home treatment teams (also known as crisis resolution teams)[6] have evolved from services developed in the 1980s and 1990s in the USA, Australia and the UK. However, as with all the new teams described in this section, the research base is for an approach which appears to combine assertive community treatment, home treatment and, to some degree, early intervention, although the latter does have its own literature to support it.

What are they?

Home treatment teams provide precisely what their name says, treatment in the client's own home which includes providing additional short-term support to clients in supported accommodation, group homes or hostels. The term has recently become synonymous with services providing intensive support – i.e. at least daily contact – as an alternative to admission to hospital.

Home treatment can be provided as a function of most types of CMHT, such as those established to focus on early intervention, assertive outreach, rehabilitation or the local community, depending on the resources available to them. Services are more effective if they provide 24-hour, seven-day a week cover but emergency out of hours teams may be able to supplement daytime services. However, the latter are often established to respond to emergencies rather than to monitor, support and prevent development of crisis or manage higher levels of risk in the community. They are also limited in their ability to provide access to services outside working hours, which has been expressed as a major concern by clients. Dedicated home treatment teams have therefore been developed internationally. Basically these are teams with sufficient staff to provide a rostered service around the clock and varied experience – nurses, social workers, doctors, occupational therapists and psychologists with support and administrative staff – to provide input in the home. They may be the 'gateway' (or barrier!) to inpatient services, acting as an assessment filter to ensure that admissions occur only when other community alternatives have been explored and either found to be unsuitable, ineffective or unacceptable, or when the risks are too great to manage in these settings.

There are overlaps between different approaches to clients, for example, assertive outreach does appear to have an impact on maintaining people in their own homes, but it is probably having most impact on clients who have received little community service in the past, although they may have received quite a lot of care in acute and secure wards, prisons and homeless accommodation. Home treatment teams, where they have been established, are probably impacting most on those with severe mental health problems, substance misuse or no mental health problems at all. For the latter two groups, the more intensive community assessment process identifies people who have substance misuse as a primary diagnosis and for whom brief unplanned admissions are, if anything, harmful and certainly disruptive to them and others around them. It is also worth identifying people who may be acutely distressed but for whom alternatives to admission are much the better option. Admission can be damaging in terms of its effect on self-esteem, self-perceived coping abilities and directly from the adverse environment in many units. This screening process is therefore very valuable in ensuring admission is only occurring where necessary.

Who needs home treatment?

Home treatment has been developed primarily as an alternative to admission. Given the pressure on hospital beds, their expense and the expressed preference by most users of services to receive care based in their own homes, this will be the priority. However, there is a case for home treatment to be used for intensive therapy where admission is not considered an option. Users who can potentially benefit from intensive work with them in the home include those who are:

- agoraphobic;
- or have delusions of reference;
- or are very depressed and amotivated.

Daily visiting in particular can enable them to make progress in a way not possible without such sustained input. Regular support at home may also allow respite for carers who are then able to leave the home, or allow themselves to leave the home. There should be a continuum established, as resources allow, between local mental health teams and home treatment input.

Generally the questions to ask regarding the suitability of home treatment are:

- If the service were unavailable, would this person need hospital admission?
- Can they be supported by the team safely and effectively without such admission?

What home treatment should be offered?

Assessment continues after the initial phase where a decision is made about offering care and it is likely that further valuable information will emerge. Monitoring will be offered – but what does that mean? It can seem rather sinister – 'checking up on me'. How is it done?

- It should be a combination of listening and observation: what's happened since we last met and particularly since you last met one of the team?

- Discussion needs to be about social events as well as symptom occurrence and medication issues.
- What impact have those events had or will have?
- Discuss any key problems and progress or otherwise.
- Symptoms are important to discuss – are they worsening or improving?
- Have any new symptoms emerged?
- What about basic functions – sleep or appetite? How are they?
- How do you feel?
- How are you getting on with medication? This can easily become a source of conflict (see Chapter 3).

Observation needs to be made of expressions of mental state – signs of anxiety, agitation, confusion, anger or depression. Essentially, continuing reassessment will go on (see Chapter 2). Observation of the environment can allow detection of incipient crises by looking for changes that may be relevant such as neglect or signs of a lot of money being spent. Observations of the carer can be informative: how are they coping?

Therapy may be relevant and possible, including non-directive listening to engage with the client, problem-solving and cognitive behaviour therapy.

The types of crises encountered can include all those described elsewhere in this book.

Assertive outreach/community treatment teams

The research on assertive outreach has been highly influential in the development of services. As a concept it has found general acceptance but there has been more controversy over whether it should be applied as part of a general service (e.g. as in the Department of Health's Care Programme approach)[7] or as specific teams (according to the original Program for Assertive Community Treatment developed in Wisconsin, USA). There has also been debate about the applicability of the US model to the UK and other health systems and the nature of the health systems have meant that differences exist although, given that the issues encountered with clients are much the same, similarities are more common.

What is assertive outreach?

Assertive outreach is simply a description of a way of taking a less passive response to service delivery than has been traditional in most mental health services, involving follow-up with clients in their own homes and neighbourhoods, thus reducing the likelihood of them defaulting from services. This style of approach has been advocated by the English Department of Health since at least 1990 as part of the Care Programme approach. Despite this, the use of such an approach remained the exception rather than the rule throughout the 1990s and the development and dissemination of the Program for Assertive Community Treatment in the USA and assertive outreach teams in the UK as a consequence of the NHS Plan[8] was the result. These teams maintain high staff member to client caseload ratios (usually under 10:1), provide cover out of hours and tend to maintain team knowledge of clients so that reliance on one individual care coordinator does not compromise follow-up.

What does it do?

Assertive outreach is appropriate for clients who do not reliably attend outpatient or clinic appointments or avoid organised home visits, and who frequently do not collaborate with services or treatments[9] because they:

- have practical difficulties (e.g. financial problems, homelessness);
- are too disorganised;
- are too unwell;
- are unwilling;
- are substance misusing;
- are vulnerable to being 'led astray' or exploitation;
- have a combination of these problems.

Assertive outreach involves going to the client rather than expecting them to come to you, and working to develop a relationship which allows collaborative assessment and management. Often the focus is on helping the client manage social problems, and this may involve doing practical tasks with them, even for them, or at least arranging for them to be done, acting and advocating for them as well as working with them to reduce or cope with symptoms through the use of medication and psychological therapies. Taking medication can be a problematic issue with clients often having very negative views about it. Working with this can be key to effective intervention, recovery from this crisis and prevention of the next.

Crises with clients who are being supported by assertive outreach teams tend to be those related to significant social problems, substance misuse, behavioural presentations and psychosis, or, often, a combination of these factors. Depression and anxiety can also be important and remediable issues but may be neglected because other issues seem more significant, whereas paranoia, voices and substance misuse, for example, may be responses to such causes of distress. The influence of dual or more diagnoses needs to be considered and their interaction can make resolution of crises particularly complex. Engagement issues are often underlying factors which need to be considered and developing collaboration over treatment issues and a focus on developing an effective trusting relationship can be more than just a foundation to work from and become therapeutic in its own right. Feeling that you are not totally alone in the world and that there are people on your side trying to help you resolve the problems you see around you can have a major effect on what seems like a crisis.

The team approach that assertive outreach teams tend to take to their client group makes it very much easier to prevent and manage crises as all team members are likely to have a prior knowledge of the client and their particular social circumstances; initial assessment and engagement has already happened. The practitioner, hearing of the crisis, knows the background and it is only the more recent circumstances that need exploration.

Assertive outreach teams tend to deal with crises themselves unless they request an assessment for compulsory admission. If the home treatment team acts as a gateway to hospital beds the outreach team may need to liaise with them over alternatives to admission.

Early intervention services

Early intervention has been an aim of local mental health teams since they were first established, but work with current clients has inevitably taken precedence. However, early intervention can begin as soon as a crisis is identified and management commenced. The carer, client or referrer may not be considering longer-term issues when they present but this can nevertheless be a window of opportunity to make a major difference. The situation may not seem to be a 'crisis' but the consequences of mismanagement are such that designating it as one may be appropriate.

Early intervention is relevant for all mental disorders for which effective interventions exist and will be described in a broad context. Early treatment may reduce distress, disability and even death (from suicide in particular), although varying evidence exists on its effectiveness in improving outcomes.

What is early intervention?

Early intervention involves providing services when they are first needed and likely to be effective. The primary reason for this is that the distress and disability that so many clients and carers experience should be alleviated or at least reduced as soon as possible. This may also have an effect on the longer-term outcome of the problem.

Early intervention has traditionally been focused on early detection and management of depression, and more recently teams have been established to work with psychosis. The principles and much of the practice applies across diagnostic categories. However, a major issue is how to identify clients likely to benefit from early intervention. Primary care has been a particular focus for this with some success in the detection of depression. However, even established services only estimate that they reach a minority of people who eventually go on to have psychotic illnesses. Orientating services towards early intervention requires similar changes to those involved in preventing and responding to crises. Detecting early signs of psychosis in those presenting for the first time is the focus but it is also important to do so in those who have had other diagnoses. Many clients who are eventually given a diagnosis of psychosis initially present and may be managed with an alternative diagnosis of drug misuse, borderline personality disorder or depressive illness.

What can early intervention teams do?

As discussed, early intervention teams usually target people with emerging psychotic symptoms but early intervention should apply to any potentially severe mental health problem. The most important justification for it is that services which can alleviate distress and disability should be made available as soon as possible to those who need them. From a service perspective, there is some justification for targeting emergence of psychotic illness as this is particularly likely to present late. With psychosis, the trigger for intervention tends to be potential positive symptoms, especially where combined with vulnerability (e.g. a shy or very sensitive personality, schizoid or paranoid), a family history, increasing social withdrawal or generally deteriorating performance. Such negative symptoms may be the main focus of concern but tend to be identified late as signs of emerging illness. With possible bipolar disorder, the emergence of disinhibition and impulsivity which is out of keeping with normal behaviour may be the signal for involvement. With other disorders, the point at which early intervention by mental health services is appropriate may be more difficult to determine. With depression, such intervention is likely to be after first-line measures in primary care have been used, and with anxiety after basic counselling and self-help, friends and problem-solving have been tried. If psychotic symptoms or risk issues are emerging, earlier intervention may be appropriate.

Terminology can be fraught with difficulties and be very disengaging. Schizophrenia is the classic example of a term which has become negatively associated with violence and poor outlook. It is one that patients frequently reject or feel very uncomfortable for this reason. Introduction of the term can change a discussion with the individual and family into a fraught crisis. Terms like spastic, Mongol, retard, even manic depressive have all been successfully replaced with other terms. It is not the case that the underlying illness is such that any change will immediately become as stigmatised as much as the previous one. Changes in such terms to cerebral palsy, Down's syndrome, learning disability and bipolar disorder have been much more acceptable to individuals and carers although not, of course, eliminating the associated stigmatisation. Terms such as drug-related psychosis, (post) traumatic (stress) psychosis, anxiety psychosis and (stress) sensitivity disorder or alternatively Bleuler's syndrome[10] are examples which have been introduced to circumvent the problems that arise with current terminology. More general symptom-based terms can be helpful such as 'voice hearer', nervous break-down, even paranoia. Collaboration with appropriate treatment regimes, whether psychosocial or pharmacological, is the goal and it is important not to let terminology get in the way.

Loss of job, friends and self-respect commonly occurs when people experience mental health problems and remedial action at an early stage is much more likely to minimise long-term damage. The person often makes decisions about these areas when ill which have unconsidered long-term consequences. It is worth identifying current meaningful activity, such as work, education or leisure, and consider these as part of crisis plans with the aim of maintaining them:

- for work, this may mean contact and negotiation with employers or education providers;
- for friendships, establishing who the current friends are and then working out how to maintain contact is important;
- self-respect and respect of others needs identifying as an issue early and appropriate education used.

So, for work, there may be contact and negotiation with employers or education providers to allow time off for full recovery. Jobs or courses can be held open if employers are aware of timescales, or promises can be extracted to reconsider the person for the position or a similar one later. It may even be that simply getting a written reference at this point will assist later on. For the client, continuing social contact with work may be helpful – although it is important not to pressurise and that the person and their family do not maintain unrealistic expectations. Conversely, staff usually have expectations that are too low. Return to work does not necessarily require remission of symptoms.

For friendships, establishing early on who the current or recent circle of friends are and then working out how to maintain contact is important. Where social contact is difficult currently, ensuring that friends have appropriate information is useful. Families will often do this but may need encouragement and advice on what to say.

Self-respect and respect of others needs identifying as an issue early on – explanation of mental health problems and information about them can help here. Identifying if the person is blaming themselves or seeing themselves as inadequate makes it possible to use appropriate analogies to help maintain their self-respect. The description of mental health problems as an illness can be tricky, as it can imply that only physical treatments are important and that a passive response to being treated is the most appropriate one. Neither of these assumptions is correct with physical illness or mental health problems.

Early work on reducing self-blame can have enduring positive effects on the individual's attitudes and those of their family and friends. Developing acceptable and understandable explanations that can be used to describe what has happened to the client can improve relationships significantly (role-playing or at least verbalising responses to situations can be very useful: 'So, what would you say if you met a workmate in the street who asked what had been happening to you?').

Carers can provide invaluable information and need the opportunity to provide it (see Chapter 2). Where a decision is made to intervene, providing the client with information, taking into account confidentiality issues (see Chapter 3) is likely to be helpful to all concerned. Where intervention is not thought to be appropriate, careful explanation of why it is not needed should be given. An explanation for the behaviour, where it is not thought to be due to significant mental health problems, is useful. For example:

- he/she may be stressed by exams, or falling out with friends, etc;
- he/she may be behaving like this because you aren't getting on too well together at the moment – as often happens in adolescence;
- this may be his/her way of beginning to develop his/her own adult identity – sometimes people push those close to them away so that they can become more confident and independent.

With any early intervention it is important to provide specific times for follow-up, and a contact name and number for the client or their carer to use if the situation should change. Communication with the original referrer of decisions is also important.

Perinatal teams

These are services set up to met the mental health needs of pregnant women and those who have just had babies. They would usually aim to identify women during pregnancy if there is a pre-existing severe mental health problem or history of problems perinatally. For new presentations they would work with a client until her problem was resolved or, for example, until the baby was a year old, whichever comes sooner. The service addresses the mental health problems associated with childbirth:

- 'baby blues' is very common, typically peaking in the fifth day after the birth and then resolving; however it can persist or deepen to become depression requiring intervention, days or weeks later;
- psychosis, usually mania/hypomania (but can be onset or relapse of schizophrenia) can develop rapidly and risks to self or child need consideration.

These teams can also help with any other mental health problem a client may have, unrelated to pregnancy. Pregnancy and becoming a parent are enormously stressful times and this raises vulnerability to mental distress. Clients with pre-existing mental health problems may have had to change or even stop medication during pregnancy and old coping strategies may become obsolete as a result of the extreme life changes that childbirth involves, so the risk of relapse is heightened.

What do perinatal teams do?

Inpatient and outpatient perinatal care may be needed for pregnant women and mothers who want their babies with them. Community provision may include mental health nurses or social workers as well as medical staff with good links to midwives, health visitors and children and family services. Group work can also be a feature as women can get peer support with managing their problems. A crèche can often be provided.

Teams like this often work by providing expert advice to other mental health services who are working with the client. Perinatal teams are able to advise about medication and possible interventions for clients known to other mental health services without taking the responsibility of care away from the team that already knows the client.

As with many of the smaller specialist teams, a perinatal team is likely to pick up a crisis presentation if it involves a client they already know. If there is a crisis presentation for a new client then much depends on local policy as to who picks up the referral. Some teams have the resources to be able to take referrals in crisis directly from general practice, a health visitor or any other mental health team that has taken the information. This is the ideal scenario for clients. Teams who cannot do this should be able to offer advice to colleagues from other teams who are assessing women in these situations and say if they are likely to be able to offer the follow-up support required.

Access to any inpatient facilities should always be negotiated in crisis presentations and use of mother and baby mental health units is usually preferred by, and is better for, clients to general inpatient care.

Use of medication in pregnancy, especially during first three months and after childbirth, needs careful consideration and expert advice. In principle, the less medication taken the less risk of harm to the newborn, however where there is a previous history of depressive illness, bipolar disorder or psychosis, this can also cause risks, including of relapse, which need to be considered. It may be that the mother will need to be advised not to breastfeed but as this can affect the relationship with their baby and their own mood, it is not advice to give lightly.

Guidance about specific drugs should always be sought from an expert source, however:

- Anti-psychotics can have adverse effects but may be needed. There is data on older drugs such as Chlorpromazine and Trifluoperazine suggesting that risks are low; emerging data on Clozapine and Olanzepine suggest a low risk of gestational diabetes and, along with Risperidone and Quetiapine, there is little evidence of malformations.

- Abrupt discontinuation of mood stabilisers is associated with rapid relapse but use of Lithium, Carbamazepine and Valproate is relatively contraindicated in pregnancy because of association with malformations.
- Use of tricyclics is well established and there are low risks to the newborn associated.
- Fluoxetine seems a relatively safe anti-depressant in pregnancy. Shorter-acting drugs such as Paroxetine or Venlafaxine may cause discontinuation symptoms in the newborn (e.g. agitation and irritability, even convulsions). Psychosocial treatments might be worth considering as first-line management.
- Benzodiazepines are best avoided.

Recommendations for women who are breastfeeding are:

- anti-depressants: Paroxetine or Sertraline;
- anti-psychotics: Sulpiride or Olanzepine;
- mood stabilisers: avoid if at all possible, Valproate if essential;
- sedatives: Lorazepam for anxiety, Zolpidem for sleep.

Eating disorders services

These are specialist teams that work with people suffering from eating disorders, usually meaning anorexia and bulimia. While there may be clients who have aspects of these disorders as part of their presentation the specialist service is likely to work with clients for whom eating problems are the *main* issue. They sometimes have dedicated inpatient beds and these are often necessary when risks warrant admission. Liaison with general medical teams may be necessary for refeeding when weight loss is profound. The crisis issues arising are described in Chapter 8, although other decisions and dilemmas faced may be informed by discussions in relation to self-harm, anxiety, depression and obsessions.

Drug and alcohol teams

Most areas have access to specialist services for people with drug and alcohol problems, comprising nurses, psychiatrists, psychologists, counsellors and social workers. Non-statutory services have become increasingly involved in providing services in this area, with counselling and advice (Alcohol Advisory Services) and support (Alcoholics Anonymous). Teams will usually provide community detoxification support and have access to admission facilities where necessary. Some provide day services and longer-term residential care. Overlap with other services occurs commonly and can be difficult – substance misuse co-morbidity is very common. Joint discussion, training and working together can help resolve these issues long-term but in the immediate crisis can be difficult. Risk minimisation is often a more realistic goal than abstinence but this judgement needs to be made by experienced staff. In these circumstances, determining what effective interventions are likely to be successful can be a joint decision. For example, it can be very difficult to help someone who is depressed and drinking heavily until they have significantly decreased their alcohol intake; on the other hand sometimes a combined approach to someone who is using cannabis to cope with voices can successfully deal with both issues. Sometimes where substance misuse is persistent and unresponsive to interventions, agreement between teams that this is the case with subsequent discussion with the client and often communication with carers and involved agencies (including family doctor) may necessitate withdrawal of service until the client is ready to effectively re-engage. The steps the client needs to take to re-engage and the supports available for carers need to be clearly defined.

Rehabilitation/resettlement teams

As the mental hospitals began to be replaced by community accommodation in the 1960s and 1970s, most services developed resettlement teams to assist clients during this transitional period and eventually many of these converted to become rehabilitation teams. These teams offer a service to clients with mental health problems who need long-term support to be able to manage in the community, especially those with symptoms of psychosis that are recurrent and interfere significantly with their lives. These teams have in many areas been going through further transition and some have converted to assertive outreach functions or merged with CMHTs.

An aim of most rehabilitation teams is to avoid crises occurring for team clients by providing effective support and prompt access to it. However, where crises arise, they provide crisis management, as described elsewhere, at times with the support of other teams and facilities (e.g. home treatment and inpatient settings). Maintaining clients in their own accommodation, at least in the crisis, is usually an aim, with review of their needs at a later stage.

As in all mental health settings, paradoxically the avoidance of the possibility that crisis can occur has meant that clients are sometimes held back from moving forward towards recovery and more independent living. Low expectations of abilities to cope have limited referrals for employment and self-supporting accommodation where clients themselves may prefer to take the risk of relapse to improve their quality of life.[11] Some rehabilitation teams have tried to counter this by actively promoting recovery in their client group rather than focusing solely on the long-term nature of their clients' problems. Many do this by working towards social inclusion, for example by organising groups to watch the local football team, or visits to sports venues, and accompanying and encouraging clients in activities of their choosing. The creative use of support workers in rehabilitation teams can offer clients a choice between services set up for people with mental health problems or accessing community facilities. This can offer effective support to those people with long-term problems who may have family responsibilities or who wish to take up voluntary work as a first step back to paid employment. There may be more formal work going on in rehabilitation teams, either cognitive therapy for psychosis or structured family work, or work on clients' own plans for recovery and how they would define and achieve this.

The move away from the long-stay hospital system meant that there were a large number of clients who had led quite (or very) institutionalised lives and rehabilitation teams catered well for this group. In more recent times, they have had to change to offer services to younger people coming into the service with psychosis in the main, including many who misuse substances. This has presented challenges as services appropriate to younger people can be radically different to those enjoyed by more mature clients. It has also led to new forms of structured work such as awareness of how drug use affects symptoms in positive and negative ways. Newer medications with less debilitating side-effects have offered greater life opportunities to clients who need medication long term, and rehabilitation teams can be active in promoting this by giving access to skills that lead to employment or other fuller social inclusion such as confidence-building and social skills training.

General hospital liaison teams

Liaison psychiatry, sometimes known as consultation-liaison or psychological medicine is an area of mental health care that primarily focuses on work with clients in general hospitals or attending specialist medical clinics (e.g. renal or rheumatology clinics). Referrals tend to be from these settings rather than from CMHTs and other teams although they may be able to offer expert advice. Liaison psychiatry's role in responding to crises varies. In areas with smaller general hospitals or with small liaison teams, this work may well fall to CMHTs and the psychiatrists attached to them. Crises can certainly arise in general hospitals, involving physical presentations of psychiatric problems, stress reactions and risk issues. Communication with medical and nursing staff will be particularly important in management.

Interface issues

Crises often raise issues of responsibility for provision of assessment and continuing services. Crises may even be *caused* by such issues where services are unilaterally withdrawn or disputes between service members arise. Such problems can be prevented by developing agreed protocols which clearly define:

- where responsibility lies;
- how transfers should occur;
- which teams also provide shared services where this may be appropriate.

The key determinant should be the needs of the individual client but these have to be balanced by considerations of how best to provide a service to the population as a whole. For example, a woman of 67 in part-time employment who has become depressed for the first time might be best served by adult rather than old-age services. A young man of 20 who has never worked, is living at home with parents and is presenting after a family crisis might be assessed as likely to benefit from family work, career advice and links with education services that a child and adolescent service can provide. However, provision of services could become chaotic if such a course was regularly followed. Extending the age range to 70 for adult services might make sense, although moving that of children's' services to 20 probably wouldn't. Consideration of such issues in protocols building in defined flexibility can assist in crisis situations. Arguments between service teams undoubtedly worsen crises and can lead, indeed have led, to catastrophes.

Old-age services have greater experience in dealing with dementias and their assistance in assessing and then taking on management of them is generally appropriate for the individual and services. However, younger patients with dementia may be difficult to nurse in old-age wards and accommodation so assistance from adult services may be needed under shared care arrangements. Alternatively, older people who are in employment and physically fully active may benefit from community supports that adult services are aware of and have access to. Adolescents who have left school and are at least potentially seeking employment, especially where they have developed mental health problems which are likely to require support and management well into adult life (e.g. psychotic illnesses), may benefit from early transfer to adult services. Collaboration between adult and adolescent services in early intervention can also share skills and access to facilities effectively.

If a client is already working with a particular service, if they experience a problem, whether of crisis proportions or not, they will normally contact the people they know and who support them. Those practitioners are best placed to manage the situation. However, there are times when the interface between services causes difficulties:

- When a person is not allocated to a service. This becomes worse for a client who may have been formerly working with a team and has had their 'case' closed. The client contacts say, an early intervention or a perinatal team in need of help, but gets sent back to their family doctor

who is told to ring the CMHT. Where services are stretched, there can be lengthy discussions about which service should take the client and this can lead to the client being passed around the system, which in turn increases both distress and risk. A client can end up being assessed by several teams before being accepted by one, which is wasteful of resources and disrespectful to the client, who has had to tell their story repeatedly.
- Where a person is allocated to a team and the allocated worker or duty worker wishes to enlist another team's support to manage a crisis. In reality, the teams that the practitioner will want are likely to be the home treatment service or the inpatient team, though it can be the case that requests for joint assessments with other teams are made. The interface problems here come if the other teams do not accept the assessment of the allocated worker. Either the original practitioner is left having to put in place a plan which is not the one indicated by their assessment or the client has to be assessed again by the other team which makes the original worker's assessment a waste of time.

The issues here are essentially about criteria for acceptance to a particular service and how advice can be readily accessed from other services. There are two principles to start from in examining how to improve interface disputes when supporting people in crisis:

- we should *all* be interested in helping the client requesting assistance;
- we should wish to avoid the client having multiple assessments, for the sake of their well-being and for the sake of limited mental health resources.

No system can ever be perfect but the following guidelines could help the process:

- if each team has a clear statement about their criteria for acceptance which they then stick to (unless the person needs help but falls in the gap between the different service criteria);
- if a client meets the criteria for a team (such as for home treatment) that team accepts a triage-style assessment from the referring team to avoid duplication or else does a joint assessment where eligibility for the service is in question;
- duty workers in all teams are trained in triage assessment, knowing what information to get over the phone to pass on;
- all teams have somebody available to offer advice on their particular specialist area to colleagues from other teams seeking help in a crisis.

Chapter 10

Preventing crises

When we discussed the nature of mental health crises and their assessment in Chapters 1 and 2, we looked at how an individual's own response to distress interacted with their social environment and support systems and also with the social, economic and political issues in the wider community. Here we take the same approach to preventing mental health crises. Bad, unpleasant things happen in life. There is no way of eliminating hazards from the world around us or of making ourselves impervious to distress. Clients may have unrealised potential, but sometimes avoid any possibility of a crisis. This can be more harmful in the long term than risking a crisis occurring and dealing with it.

Prevention of crises has to begin with the first crisis with which the client presents. How a person is supported and the approach taken is going to influence future coping strategies. It may be that the client and carer learn skills and develop a plan for future difficulties through the first crisis presentation. It may also be the case that they do not. Crises do reach a resolution but the intervention may not have prepared the client for future problems, particularly if there was a barrier to engagement with the client, such as a compulsory admission or no continuity of professional staff involvement. So although intervening in a mental health crisis carries the seeds for future prevention, there is also a need to focus on this sort of prevention work when doing the follow-up work with clients who have found their feet again and are receiving community support.

There are four aspects to this work:

1 Individual crisis prevention planning: work with clients on their own trigger points, symptom management and vulnerabilities; finding ways to maximise coping.
2 Work with clients on looking at the possibilities of changing those parts of their social situation that are making them more vulnerable to poor mental health.
3 Look for and support improvements in community facilities that promote good mental health.

4 Campaign for social and political change that is socially inclusive and supports clients to use the good policies that are in place such as anti-discriminatory legislation (e.g. the Disability Discrimination Act in the UK).

Individual crisis prevention planning

In many services, a crisis prevention plan is drawn up with clients known to mental health teams. However, these frequently emphasise what the client wants to happen when the crisis is already upon them rather than preventing it happening. Also they tend to be completed in quite a cursory way with little real detail. A client may choose to have a very brief plan and that is fine. However, it may be because this part of the 'paperwork' is completed quickly with the client being put on the spot at multi-disciplinary reviews – being asked to give a view there and then about what they find helpful. This is likely to continue for as long as review procedures are seen as meetings rather than as a continuing process.

In reality, plans to prevent crises and minimise the harmful effects of relapse can constitute a substantial piece of work done jointly with the client and quite possibly with their carers too. Even when a client wants to keep it brief, it needs dedicated time put aside to be done properly. Recovery is a very individual concept and does not necessarily equate with being symptom-free. The client's own values and wishes about where they want to be in life and what route they take to get there have to be at centre stage in negotiating these plans.

What is helpful in a prevention plan?

- What keeps the person well? This can serve as a reminder to the client to do some of these things. Examples might include 'not isolating myself', 'taking medication' or 'having relaxation time'.
- What could be potential triggers for worsening symptoms? Again this is highly individual, for example, drinking too much alcohol, seeing an abusive relative, worry about anything without sharing it, doing too much. To make these meaningful some tips on how to avoid or manage the triggers can be included which may just involve doing more of the things that keep the person well or may involve a new coping strategy like phoning a friend or a mental health worker.
- Early warning signs are fundamental to a crisis prevention plan and might include the beginning or worsening of symptoms. Some people for example know that poor sleep or a loss of energy are indicators that worse may come. It is at this stage that a plan needs to be put into action. However, it is also important that early signs which are quite non-specific do not lead to an overreaction from client and carer – a couple of

nights' poor sleep or a brief episode of voices does not mean inevitable deterioration.

What helps? This can include symptom management and social support. It can include such instructions to self as 'ring my mum', 'take an extra tablet as we agreed', 'use relaxation tape', 'tell care coordinator' or 'practise mindfulness techniques'. Some of what helps is about personal preference and can relate to the client's social support. However, there are some ways of coping that are symptom-specific and it is important that practitioners help clients to acquire new skills that they can use when times get hard. Part of prevention is trialling out these techniques in not so bad times to find out what works for the client and what does not. There are many useful publications that can assist staff to advise clients on ways to manage voices, coping with anxiety, lifting their mood or managing emotional coping difficulties.[1] There are also some self-help books that are useful (see notes 3 and 5 in Chapter 5).

Drugs and talk

Medication has an established role in preventing relapse in depression, bipolar disorder and schizophrenia. For depression, evidence for its use for six months after an initial episode in reducing the likelihood of recurrence is good. Where repeated episodes have occurred, the case is quite good for continuing use over much longer periods, although the studies needed to demonstrate that this is actually effective are few. Mood stabilisers such as Lithium and Valproate, and some anti-psychotics, such as Olanzepine and Quetiapine, reduce relapse of mania although they are less effective against depression with side-effects longer-term that need to be considered. Anti-psychotics reduce relapse in schizophrenia in many patients but collaboration can be an issue (see Chapter 3).

Talk can also help. Social support will be discussed more fully below. Psychological intervention has been demonstrated to reduce relapse in depression, anxiety, schizophrenia, bulimia and possibly mania. It may also reduce self-harm rates in borderline personality disorder. Such therapies therefore need to be considered as part of the crisis plan. Self-help books can be a first step, as discussed above. Computerised cognitive behaviour therapy programmes[2] and websites are available and can allow at least familiarisation with the techniques. Referral for psychological assessment will be relevant to many people – as many as medication is relevant for – but availability is likely to continue to be limited in many areas, with trained workforce shortages for some time. The potential for assertive outreach of psychological services, booster work and longer-term effective interventions in crisis prevention is considerable but unlikely to be met until a major shift in resources occurs.

Role of advance directives

Some people may choose to formalise their views about their future care and record an advance directive. These can be valuable in articulating the view of the client about the care they want to receive, or not receive when they are in crisis, and may not be able to say this clearly for themselves. Such directives are not legally binding but professionals should take them into account when considering options for care. Advance directives are limited in relation to prevention because they tend to focus on what to do when a crisis is reoccurring rather than how the person can stay free of symptoms or maintain manageable symptoms.

The format of a plan

Some people have a complex and well-constructed plan that is very explicit. A good example of this is the wellness recovery action plan (WRAP) that can be done in a group with peer support or by an individual with or without their care coordinator. There are forms that can be used and the recommendation is that a client uses a leaf binder so that decisions can be updated. As well as their WRAP, clients can have a 'wellness toolbox' and a 'post-crisis plan'. Further information is available from www.mentalhealthrecovery.com.

Less extensive documentation is available as part of most review forms or a client can make their own using a format or language that is theirs. Flow charts suit some people while for people who are less happy with the written word, audio-taping can be of more use.

Who is the plan shared with?

This is up to the client but it makes sense for them to share the existence and broad content of the plan with anybody named as having a role to play. If a client names a particular friend as being the person who will be supportive, that person will need to know what the client wants them to do or not to do. Inclusion prominently in clinical records or with duty teams, ideally on networked computer systems or ready for faxing, can make sure that the plan is available when it is needed – often out of working hours and not necessarily on mental health premises. It is sensible to prominently include the plan in clinical records and for it to be accessible to duty or out-of-hours teams.

Problem-solving life stresses

Many clients face life stresses that even if not directly contributing to their mental health issues certainly can make matters worse. The discussion about individual coping strategies and skills we have already had is relevant to managing life stresses, but a client may need support to get over seemingly impossible hurdles before they can gain confidence in their own abilities to cope. For example, in working with a depressed man who is at risk of eviction from his home, there is little point working out with him how to manage worsening symptoms to prevent a crisis without also arming him with legal and financial advice and with the support and skills to access these essential services.

While we focus on supporting people to be able to cope in mental health services, there is often a parallel fear of fostering dependence. Independence and individual coping skills are certainly important but we live in a society and are inevitably dependent on each other for help. Some clients get the message or else believe that they should always go it alone. In fact, asking for and using the help and support of others is a set of skills for clients to learn and institute as part of the recovery process. There is also the bare fact that at times practitioners see people who are just too disabled by their mental health problems at that point in time to be able to do very urgent tasks. It is part of the duty of care to offer assistance in these instances. In fact, what clients often value over other input is practical help and support. Being helpful to clients or immediately arranging help can be a critical part of engagement with the client in the early stages of working together. Often, particularly with clients who have long-standing dependency needs, the only way forward is to provide sufficient support to allow them to build the skills and the confidence to begin to stand on their own.

The issues that may be affecting service users are hugely varied and practitioners will never have all the answers. What practitioners do need is a set of skills and sufficient administration time to undertake the telephone calls and letter-writing involved in giving practical assistance with social issues.

The sorts of skills needed include being able to:

- enable the client to name the worries that they have;
- be a bit of a private detective – a co-investigator;
- obtain a knowledge base that covers the fundamentals of the most common issues that are likely to arise;
- use skills of support as required;
- use advocacy skills;
- be aware of the additional support and practical help that people may need.

Enabling the client to name their worries

Some clients sit on appalling problems because they are scared of facing them, are in denial, and fear that verbalising them will make them unable to cope. They fear that their anxieties will be belittled or that they will be judged negatively by staff if they admit to whatever is on their mind. These quite understandable fears can be minimised by staff that show a non-judgemental attitude, who ask empathic questions about social issues while offering reassurance that practical life problems are a frequent feature of mental distress and help is often available. A skilled worker can tell people that naming a problem does not make it worse. When issues around the client involve concerns about children, staff need to be sensitive to and clear about the limits of confidentiality, the needs and rights of the children and the fact that children's social services do not just go around removing children – they do actually work towards helping families to manage problems and live happier lives.

Being a private detective

The most experienced practitioner will still come across new problems and the skill is to find out who or what is available to help the client. We discussed community mapping in Chapter 2, and having access to local information is invaluable here. The use of contacts, making telephone calls and having internet access are also ways of tracking down organisations or sources of knowledge that are of use.

Obtaining a knowledge base

Being able to obtain a knowledge base is very important. Community mental health practitioners need as a minimum a working knowledge of the welfare benefits system, local housing provision, local drugs and alcohol services, local advice centres, rape crisis centres and domestic violence helplines, plus service information. Benefits awareness is particularly important. Issues concerning money are not just about relieving immediate worries. We know that 'the positive association between poverty and mental health problems is one of the best established in all of psychiatric epidemiology'.[3] Having the skills to pursue anti-poverty strategies with clients is crucial to recovery and preventing relapse. This involves income maximisation for clients on benefit and supporting clients to move to employment if they wish to go down this route. This work could also involve budgeting, being aware of local credit unions if they exist and knowing the cheapest local places to shop. Issues of employment and discrimination are getting more attention and practitioners need to know how to advise or refer on for help clients facing problems in this area.

Using skills of support

Using skills of support as required means the ability to communicate and negotiate with the client, as the client's needs can change from day to day. We discussed the tension between offering practical help and building self-confidence earlier, but broadly the aim of good practice has to be for the client to achieve their goals with minimum but sufficient help from services. The aim of practitioners is to encourage clients to use their own skills to sort out problems, and clients gain self-confidence and self-esteem by doing so, which in turn assists in the prevention of future problems. If practitioners underestimate how much support clients need they can push clients into situations that stress them further and confirm negative beliefs about themselves. It all boils down to listening to your client. If a very capable client is saying to you, 'I really cannot go into the benefits agency on my own today as my voices are really bad' then it is *not* fostering dependence to go with them. On the contrary, it is positive that the client is assertively asking for help and could be fed back to the client as such.

There are times when services can hold clients back by inadvertently doing too much for them, so reducing their confidence. Continuous communication and checking out with the client should minimise this risk. However, sometimes a client may feel they cannot cope but a practitioner believes they can. Confidence can be built in these cases by graded exposure to stressful situations. Staying in the background when a client is say, at the Citizens' Advice Bureau or a housing office is a step forward, letting the client lead and use their own problem-solving skills. To accompany this, clients can be encouraged to use their individual coping and stress management skills to help get themselves though the stress of a given situation.

Using advocacy skills

Being an advocate is totally different from offering support and the two are easily confused. There are likely to be times when a client is unable to do something for themselves and wishes you to advocate on their behalf. They may prefer to have access to an independent advocate which should always be a possibility open to them, but some clients prefer to ask someone they already know, so it is a role often taken on by care coordinators. In advocacy, you are presenting the client's views and wishes, not those being suggested by a staff member or carer. In decisions about debt or housing or anything in life, every individual will have their own value system. In acting as an advocate, there is a need to firstly thoroughly check out that what you are going to say is in concordance with the client's wishes – and this is an ongoing process as people have the right to change their minds. It is a skill to pass a client's wishes on to another agency without slanting what you say or write with an agenda that is not the client's. There are times when a conflict of interest can arise or you may feel uncomfortable with the role of advocate. The skill here is in recognising this and making a decision to use other advocacy services to assist the client instead.

Calling on additional support

Clients may need additional support and practical help but are excluded from mainstream services for reasons other than their mental health, and we need to be aware of this. People may feel unwelcome in services or the way services are set up may not meet their needs or may deny them access. People facing this sort of discrimination may be refugees, travellers, or people who have lower levels of literacy or a different first language to the one services use. Some research has revealed a 'lack of preventative and after care services which are appropriate for Black and ethnic minority communities'.[4] In addition, people may be excluded due to their age or sexuality. Those clients who have a physical or learning disability on top of their mental health problem face all sorts of complications. Services bat them between each other and professionals offering support with one problem may not have the knowledge and skills to help with the other. Working with the whole person has always been a challenge to compartmentalised professionals.

Role of the community in good mental health

There is plenty in the community that can contribute to causing mental health problems, not least the attitudes and prejudice people face, just for *having* a mental health problem. There exist in parallel some elements that build good mental health and therefore are preventative in nature. Service user research indicates that what they want are jobs, friends and money – i.e. they want the same as anybody else in the community – and professionals not accepting this are contributing to social exclusion and potentially maintaining difficulties. A practitioner focus on quality of life, whatever that may mean for the individual client, is going to be beneficial to mental health and therefore prevent crises. Using the strengths of the community's resources is helpful here as they will still be there long after mental health services have left the client's life.

Helping the client make the most of their community

You can assist your client by:

- mapping with them what facilities and support are available;
- getting help and support from mental health day services;
- exploring alternatives such as getting involved with a local place of worship or joining a gym;
- seeking employment services for people with mental health problems returning to work;
- helping the client build networks and social contacts;
- suggesting social skills training;
- developing new services that may be of use.

Clients may already have a wealth of knowledge about who or what is available locally for them. Alternatively, they may be living in a new area and have no idea. The community mapping process is helpful here (see Chapter 4). Once the options are presented to clients they can make a choice.

Many clients get tremendous help and support from mental health day services (see Chapter 9) as they are places where people are less likely to hold negative views about people with mental health problems. Peer support, a reintroduction to socialising and a safe place to find acceptance, meaningful occupation and have fun, are all compliments paid to such services by those using them. Conversely, some clients will not want to go down that route to meet people – sadly it is sometimes because they 'are not like them', themselves discriminating against people with similar problems to themselves. Clients also sometimes complain that they feel railroaded into attending groups by professionals on the grounds that 'it is good for them and they need to meet people'.

Some clients do not want to feel labelled or have staff influencing their leisure time and occupation, so day services are not for them. They can look at alternatives such as getting involved with a local place of worship or joining a gym. It may be that just starting to say good morning at the local shops is as far as a person wants to socialise, and others may prefer to have less social contact. If a client can be helped to define what would constitute a better quality of life for them, then steps can be taken towards this, whatever it may mean.

Many areas now have specialist services to assist people back into employment and there is plenty of evidence that work is protective of mental health. However, there need to be a few provisos to this as being made to work long hours or in a monotonous job or where subject to workplace bullying may have very negative effects. On the whole though, work provides self-esteem, better financial security, a social role and often a social life. If local employers can be advised in how to support employees via flexible working hours or a time-out place to assist in relapse prevention then skilled workers are less likely to be lost to the workplace. For some clients who had jobs prior to developing mental health problems it can be a massive upheaval to return to work, not because of their ability but because of employers' assumptions about people with mental health problems. Practitioners hear stories of people being demoted, pressured to leave or not being taken seriously as having a disability. Anti-discriminatory legislation (e.g. the Disability Discrimination Act in the UK) is helping clients, and trade unions or local legal services can be enormously helpful also.

For clients who have not worked for a long time there are bigger hurdles. The past received wisdom has been that people with severe mental health problems should not be encouraged towards the workplace. This was due to the belief that 'people with mental illness were not expected to recover'.[5] With the welcome emergence of the recovery movement and with clients moving to take control of their lives back from professionals, this assumption is being challenged. What service users may need is support to gain employment. This can mean help to get voluntary work as a stepping stone or to get a reference;

it can mean mock interviews and advice on application forms, help to learn or relearn key skills or just peer support. Some areas have services specifically for mental health clients but if there are none, or if the client prefers not to use them, then all areas (in the UK at least) have disability employment advisers at the job centre and many have general voluntary sector services for generic disability and job finding. Practitioners should get to know some of these key people who can be such a positive resource.

While employment provides money, company and social roles for people, and the consequential social inclusion can be of enormous benefit, any push from government to get people into work may be viewed by clients and practitioners with suspicion – is it about supporting recovery or to do with reducing the benefits bill in the country? Clients can find it hugely stressful when they are called in to see doctors from benefits agencies to justify their disability status, and there is a perceived pressure to conform to a new model, a sort of 'recover or else' message. There are also some jobs that can be damaging to mental health, either through the fact that they are too stressful or too monotonous or because the person is expected to work without what is termed 'reasonable adjustments' to accommodate a person's particular disability. Work is not a panacea but it should be an option. In the end social inclusion is about enabling clients to 'get a life back' and it has to be the life they want, not the one professionals think is good for them.

Helping people build networks and social contacts can be difficult, especially for people who have become isolated by their illness or for those who have moved away from the family home and are starting again. The losses associated with mental ill health are enormous. Clients may have lost their jobs, friends, suffered relationship breakdown or loss of income. In the process of recovery, there are hurdles to rebuilding the social networks that can help people get better. Common problems suffered include finding it hard to talk to anyone if having a bad day and non-sufferers not understanding this, or having to hide the problem in case people think a mental health problem makes them homicidal. It can be a slow process.

Social skills training for people who have really lost confidence can be of huge benefit. Some team occupational therapists will do this or at least provide material and advice for care coordinators. Such training involves:

- practising or role-playing social interactions to help gain confidence;
- reminding clients of their strengths;
- using any existing social outlet (e.g. family or old friends) to be supportive in going to new places;
- use of support workers, befrienders or buddies to go with clients to community activities;
- respecting the client's own value system – if the client wants to meet their social needs at the local place of worship or the local pub (or both) then that is their choice.

Most care coordinators don't have the opportunity to involve themselves in development work beyond flagging up to managers what might be of use and encouraging clients to give feedback. For those who do, examples of local initiatives might be a shared transport scheme for service users in areas poorly served by public transport, informal buddying for service users to attend a local gym or the development of a befriending service.

There is also the opportunity of getting to know your local generic resources and talking with their staff about the issues for people with mental health problems. Many services are keen to be accessible to members of the community who feel excluded and with a bit of information can consider how they present themselves or combat any bias present to make that possible. Much of this type of work happens over time as staff get to know the local areas they work in.

Politics, policy and social inclusion

This section is really an acknowledgement of the impact of the bigger picture. What is happening on an economic, cultural and political level has an impact on all citizens, so whether somebody is a client or service provider (or indeed both at the same time) it is worth being aware of the restrictions and opportunities that exist due to movements on the wider stage. We will discuss what can be achieved from being aware and what can be done to make use of the positives and work around the hurdles. These can then be considered in planning for prevention. Everything has an impact but we will mention specifically some of the policies, social norms and economic facts that will directly affect care and service provision and client's quality of life:

- economic situation;
- health care policy;
- mental health policy;
- implications of legislation;
- cultural presentation of mental health.

Whatever economic situation the country finds itself in is bound to affect the health of its citizens. It affects what is available to fund health care services and any increase in unemployment rates will be damaging to mental health. In an arena where people are discriminated against in the workplace for having a mental health problem, a period of competition for jobs is likely to leave them even more excluded. Reminding clients of this can help stop them blaming themselves for their situation. Conversely, periods of prosperity can provide opportunities for supported work placements as employers are encouraged to be more creative in attracting and retaining staff. This can be capitalised upon.

As well as the amount that a country has available for spending on health care, there can be wide variations in how money is spent and whether it goes to health as a priority. Then there is the issue of distribution within health, and mental health can end up being at the back of the queue in the competition. Quantity isn't everything but it is a fair bit of the equation. If mental health teams don't have the money they can't provide the services and certainly not with elements of choice. When money is short there is the possibility that the emphasis of work done will be on fire-fighting or managing crises without prevention work occurring. There are different ways of spending any money that is allocated. The closure of the long-stay hospitals may have been in part to save money, but services in the community have proved as costly, though hopefully they have provided a better quality of life and offered better choices to people. (Not a view shared by all, as service users moved from well-resourced long-stay hospitals to a shared house in the middle of an unwelcoming council estate may testify.) In theory at least we should all have some control over policy by way of our elected representatives and both practitioners and clients can use these if policy is seen as unfavourable.

Mental health policy has become increasingly focused on promoting balanced services and treatment options with psychosocial interventions alongside medication options, as demonstrated by the *National Service Framework for Mental Health* in England.[6] The introduction and funding of teams in the NHS Plan for early intervention, home treatment and assertive outreach is making a direct contribution to the prevention of crisis presentation. More recently, work on social exclusion and mental health is developing and may yet impact on stigmatisation and the potential improved social recovery and quality of life for clients. On the other hand, the more defensive public protection agenda of governments (e.g. around new mental health legislation)[7] has had a negative effect on public attitudes as evidenced by government surveys.[8] The positive aspect of this is that in the UK, a mental health alliance including clients, carers and professionals has developed which has already made an impact.

We have already mentioned the legislation regarding community care and mental health but there are other laws that impact on clients and practitioners that are hugely relevant. Practitioners and clients will regularly encounter laws to do with welfare rights and housing (e.g. local authorities' obligations to house people with disabilities or laws about capacity and power of attorney). Two pieces of legislation have made a particular impact in Britain in recent years: the Human Rights Act and the Disability Discrimination Act. The first has allowed clients to successfully challenge long-standing injustices in the current mental health legislation regarding the involvement of relatives against a client's wishes. The second establishes people's right not to be discriminated against on the grounds of their disability in their employment, leisure time or as receivers of services. It is proving useful to clients who are recovering and wish to return to work with reasonable adjustments to their conditions and hours to make this possible. Practitioners should try to keep abreast of changes in law and advise clients of their rights, not just when the Mental Health Act is being used but as citizens. In addition, because legislation is complex, knowing where clients can go for expert and free legal advice is essential.

The cultural presentation of mental health is an important issue. It is not just the media who are to blame for negative images of mental health problems. Slang terms for having mental health problems often double as terms of abuse in our language (e.g. nutter, psycho or basket case). Our children are therefore growing up with an implicit message that to have such health problems equates with something bad, and is synonymous with being despised and disapproved of. If we add to this the messages contained in the government's proposed mental health legislation, with its emphasis on public safety rather than client self-determination, then we can hardly blame media images alone for the stigmatisation of the mentally ill.

However, media representation has been largely negative, with people in psychological distress being portrayed as figures of fun or, more frequently, disproportionately involved in violent crime. The consequences for current and future clients are severe in that this makes it harder for people to ask for and receive the help and understanding they need. Clients will not benefit from early intervention services if they are ashamed to admit to their symptoms and the initial presentation to services is therefore more likely to be a crisis, as the opportunity for prevention work has been lost.

There have been some positive images of mental health clients in the media and these need to be applauded. Campaigns have been run by the Department of Health, the non-statutory sector and the Royal College of Psychiatrists along with many local organisations to try to combat stigma. Work in schools on the nature and large prevalence of mental health problems can work against some of the prejudice that is ingrained in our language and culture, and this essential work should be supported. Finally, if we are serious about reducing stigma we can make personal decisions to challenge prejudicial views and language when we come across it as an act of basic solidarity, whether we suffer from mental health problems ourselves or not.

Case example

Melody, age 23, the lone parent of a 3-year-old boy, Sam, presented in crisis to a family doctor with increased severity of self-harming by cutting and talking of her intention to take an overdose. Her boyfriend had recently walked out on her.

Prevention began at the time of the crisis as a plan to manage risk was put in place using her mum and a friend to look after her tablets and support from a mental health practitioner and her health visitor. Melody's sister and her son's father agreed to help with the little boy. Melody was prescribed an anti-depressant. All these actions could be used again when similar circumstances arose.

Post crisis work helped Melody learn other ways to cope with distress. She practised mindfulness techniques and snapped elastic bands on her wrists to produce discomfort to reduce cutting. She was encouraged to talk about her worries and, having disclosed some traumatic childhood abuse issues, began to seek counselling with a local voluntary agency specialising in this.

Melody was helped to claim benefits now that her partner had left. This helped her sort out her financial problems and taught her how to manage the 'system'. Her health visitor introduced her to a parent and toddler group to make new friends. She reinforced the fact that Melody had asked for and therefore got help from her family with her child when she wasn't coping and that this was the right thing to do. The mental health worker directly challenged Melody's beliefs of being a failure because she was a lone parent, looking at the skills and strengths Melody made use of to be a parent and how undervalued she, and parents like her, are in society. Meeting others in a similar position backed this up and helped her self-esteem.

Melody's crisis plan involved identifying warning signs as not sleeping, getting annoyed easily, not wanting to talk to people and feeling 'I can't cope'. At such times she was advised to ring a friend, eat something nice, be mindful, not put off doing things she was worried about, ring her family doctor or mental health team, give medication to her mum if she didn't feel safe, and put her son first. As a result, Melody found it easier to cope initially but had a difficult time when she started a relationship with a man who became abusive when he drank. She avoided the mental health team as she was embarrassed and guilty for having had him in the house with her son but did use her other supports. Her Mum contacted services and Melody was given positive feedback for having ended the relationship for her son's sake and for using informal supports. Although she cut during this period she did not contemplate suicide for more than fleeting moments and the situation was one of life difficulties rather than crisis.

Some final comments

What we have discussed here are some ideas that come from our experience, reading and research from social, psychological and medical perspectives and the views and experiences of clients, carers and colleagues that have been shared with us. In putting forward these suggestions, there will be areas we have not covered and useful proposals we have not made. There are also conflicting views between professionals about what works to help people suffering with mental distress which colleagues may wish to share with us in the future.

One of the many valuable messages that has come from the user movement is the importance of an inclusive human approach to mental health service delivery. We have attempted to acknowledge the person as a whole, with their varied rights and needs, however this inevitably reduces the possibility of proposing easy solutions. Individuals are so varied and complex that all we can ever try to do is help them to the best of our ability within often constrained circumstances and, in particular, to continue to listen and learn. We welcome any comments and ideas about what else works and wish you the very best in your practice. We leave the last word to Jake.

'What helped? People telling the truth, no-one told me the truth when I was ill before. This time they said you're ill . . . and you need to move forward.'

Notes

Introduction

1 Council of Europe, *Recommendation 2004(10) Concerning the Protection of the Human Rights and Dignity of Persons with Mental Disorder*. Adopted by the Committee of Ministers of the Council of Europe, 22 September 2004. www.coe.org, accessed 30.5.05.

2 Dattilio, F.M. and Freeman A. (eds) *Cognitive-Behavioral Strategies in Crisis Intervention*. New York: Guilford, 1994.

3 Brown, T.M., Scott, A.I.F. and Pullen, I.M., *Handbook of Emergency Psychiatry*. Edinburgh: Churchill Livingstone, 1990.

4 Kleespies, P.M. (ed.) *Emergencies in Mental Health Practice: Evaluation and Management*. New York: Guilford, 1998.

5 National Institute of Clinical Excellence, *Clinical Guidelines on Schizophrenia, Anxiety, Depression, Violence & Self-harm*. www.nice.org.uk, accessed 9.5.05.

6 Diamond, R., *Instant Psychopharmacology, 2nd edition*. New York: Norton, 2002.

7 Taylor, D., Paton, C. and Kerwin, R., *The Maudsley 2005–6 Prescribing Guidelines*, 8th edition. London: Taylor & Francis, 2005.

8 Phillips, K.A., First, M.B. and Pincus, H. (eds) *Advancing DSM: Dilemmas in Psychiatric Diagnosis*. Washington: American Psychiatric Association, 2003.

Chapter I

1 Rapoport, L., The state of crisis: some theoretical considerations, in In H.J. Parad (ed.) *Crisis Intervention: Selected Readings*, p. 24. New York: Family Service Association of America, 1965.

2 Kfir, N., *Crisis Intervention Verbatim*. London: Taylor & Francis, 1989, p. 3.

3 Golan, N. (1978), quoted in Payne M., *Modern Social Work Theory*. Basingstoke: Macmillan, 1991, pp. 104–5.

4 O'Hagan, K., *Crisis intervention in Social Services*. Basingstoke: Macmillan, 1986, p. 141.

5 Kifr, op. cit.

6 Smale, G., Tuson, G. and Statham, D., *Social Work and Social Problems*. Basingstoke: Palgrave, 2000, p. 3.

7 Kingdon, D.G. and Turkington, D., *Cognitive Therapy of Schizophrenia: Guides to Evidence-based Practice*. New York: Guilford, 2005.

8 Grucza, R.A. *et al.*, Personality and depressive symptoms: a multi-dimensional analysis, *Journal of Affective Disorders*, 74(2): 123–30.

9   Gabbard, G.O. (ed.) *Countertransference Issues in Psychiatric Treatment (Review of Psychiatry 18)*. Washington: American Psychiatric Publishing Inc., 1999.

Chapter 2

1   Department of Health, *Effective Coordination in Mental Health Services – Modernising the Care Programme Approach*. London: Department of Health, 1999.
2   Kingdon, D.G., The care programme approach, *Psychiatric Bulletin*, 18(2): 68–70.
3   Milner, J. and O'Byrne, P., *Assessment in Social Work, 2nd edition*. Basingstoke: Palgrave, 2002.
4   Department of Health and Welsh Office, *Mental Health Act 1983: Code of Practice*. London: The Stationery Office, 1999, para. 2.13.
5   Department of Health and Welsh Office, op. cit., para. 2.4.
6   Department of Health, *Mental Health Act 1983*. London: HMSO, section 135(1).
7   Smale, G. *et al.*, op. cit., p. 133.
8   Healthcare Commission, *Count me in: 2005 National Census of Inpatients in Mental Health Hospitals and Facilities in England and Wales*. London: Healthcare Commission, 2006.
9   Ferns, P., Finding a way forward: a black perspective, in Tew, J. (ed.) *Social Perspectives in Mental Health*. London: Jessica Kingsley.
10   Milner, J. and O'Byrne, P., op. cit., p. 10.
11   Elwood, P.Y., Characteristics of admissions deemed inappropriate by junior psychiatrists, *Psychiatric Bulletin*, 23: 34–7.
12   Timms, P., Stigma and homelessness, in A. Crisp (ed.) *Every Family in the Land*. London: Royal College of Psychiatrists, 2004.
13   Department of Health, *Carers Act*. London: HMSO, 1995.
14   Department of Health, *Children's Act*. London: HMSO, 1990.

Chapter 3

1   www.rcpsych.ac.uk/campaigns/pinc/index.htm.
2   Department of Health and Welsh Office, op cit.
3   Department of Health, *Mental Incapacity Act*. London: HMSO, 2005.

Chapter 4

1   Hawton, K. *et al.*, Schizophrenia and suicide: systematic review of risk factors, *British Journal of Psychiatry*, 187: 9–20.
2   Ingram, R. Towards no secrets, in A. Ryan and J. Pritchard (eds) *Good Practice in Adult Mental Health*. London: Jessica Kingsley, 2004, p. 309.
3   Department of Health, *Mental Health Act 1983*. London: HMSO, 1983.

Chapter 5

1   Linehan, M., *Skills Training Manual for Treating Borderline Personality Disorder*. New York: Guilford, 1993, p. 136.
2   Kinnerley, H., *Overcoming Anxiety*. London: Taylor & Francis, 1997; Marks, I., *Living with Fear*. Maidenhead: McGraw-Hill, 2001; Greenberger, D. and Padesky, C., *Mind over Mood*. New York: Guilford, 1995.
3   Gath, D. and Mynors-Wallis, L., Problem solving treatment in primary care, in, D.M. Clark and C. Fairburn (eds) *Science and Practice of Cognitive Behaviour Therapy*. Oxford: Oxford University Press, 1997.
4   Greenberger, D. and Padesky, C., *Mind over Mood*. New York: Guilford, 1995, p. 159.

5   Somer, E., *Food and Mood: The Complete Guide to Eating Well and Feeling Your Best*. New York: Owl Books, 1999.

Chapter 6

1   Plumb, S., Mapping the mental health consequences of childhood sexual abuse and similar experiences, in J. Tew (ed.) *Social Perspectives in Mental Health*. London: Jessica Kingsley, 2005, p.113.
2   Plumb, ibid., p.124.
3   Bateman, A. and Fonagy, P., Treatment of borderline personality disorder with psychodynamically orientated partial hospitalisation: an 18-month follow-up. *American Jornal of Psychology*, 158: 36–42.
4   Linehan, op cit., p. 64.
5   Linehan, ibid. p. 67.
6   Mayfield, D. *et al.*, The CAGE questionnaire; validation of a new alcoholism screening instrument, *American Journal of Psychology*, 131: 1121–3.

Chapter 8

1   Fairburn, C.G., *Overcoming Binge Eating*. New York: Guilford, 1995.

Chapter 9

1   Department of Health, *Mental Health Policy Implementation Guide: Community Mental Health Teams*. London: Department of Health, 2002.
2   Kingdon, D., Mental health practitioners: bypassing the recruitment bottleneck, *Psychiatric Bulletin*, 26: 328–31.
3   Department of Health, *Mental Health Policy Implementation Guide: Acute Inpatients*. London: Department of Health, 2002.
4   National Institute for Clinical Excellence, Violence: The Short-term Management of Disturbed/violent Behaviour in Psychiatric Inpatient Settings and Emergency Departments. Clinical guideline 25, 2002.
5   James, M. and Jongeward, D., *Born to Win: Transactional Analysis with Gestalt Experiments*. Cambridge: Da Capo Press, 1996.
6   Department of Health, *Mental Health Policy Implementation Guide: Crisis Resolution and Home Treatment Teams*. London: Department of Health, 2001.
7   Kingdon, D.G., The care programme approach, *Psychiatric Bulletin*, 18(2): 68–70.
8   Department of Health, *The NHS Plan*. London: Department of Health, 2001.
9   Burns, T. and Firn, M., *Assertive Outreach in Mental Health: A Manual for Practitioners*. Oxford: Oxford University Press, 2002.
10 Tyrer, P., Useful diagnoses. *British Journal of Psychiatry*, 185: 528.
11 Social Exclusion Unit, *Mental Health and Social Exclusion*. London: Office of the Deputy Prime Minister, 2004.

Chapter 10

1   Linehan, op. cit.
2   Wright, J., Computer-assisted CBT, in *Review of Psychiatry 23: Cognitive Behavior Therapy*. New York: American Psychiatric Association, 2004.
3   Williams, J., Women's mental health, in Tew, op. cit., p. 154.
4   Ferns, P., op. cit., p. 130.
5   Department of Health, *Journey to Recovery – The Government's Vision for Mental Health*. London: Department of Health, 2001, p. 24.

6   Department of Health, *National Service Framework for Mental Health*. London: Department of Health, 1999.
7   Department of Health, *Draft Mental Health Bill*. London: The Stationery Office, 2002.
8   RSGB, Attitude survey to mental illness, www.doh.gov.uk, accessed 21.05.05.

Appendix 1: Making sense

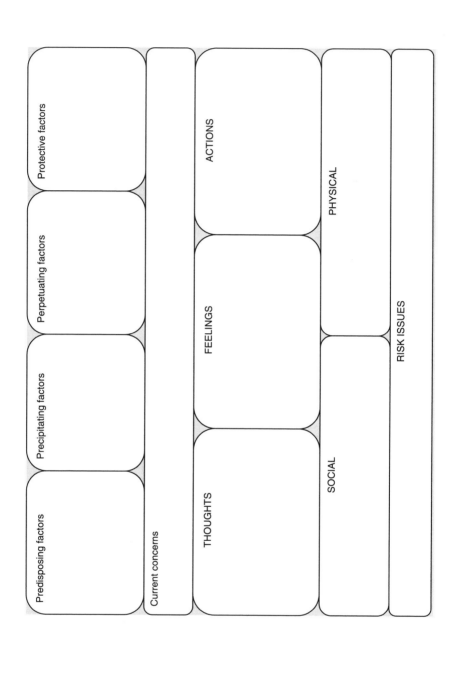

Predisposing factors

Precipitating factors

Perpetuating factors

Protective factors

Current concerns

THOUGHTS

FEELINGS

ACTIONS

SOCIAL

PHYSICAL

RISK ISSUES

Appendix 2: Anxiety pamphlet

Anxiety

This pamphlet has been written to help you to understand why we become anxious and how it affects us. It is important to understand because anxiety 'feeds' on itself. In other words, worry about the effects of anxiety itself can often increase that anxiety.

Does anxiety ever have a purpose?

Most people are familiar with the feelings of anxiety; 'butterflies' in the stomach before an interview, an examination or a date with a boy or girlfriend. The effect of this is to 'key you up' or get you 'on your toes' which means that you are alert and ready for action. You feel your muscles tense, your heart beats faster, your stomach tightens up and you concentrate on the task in front of you, trying to predict what is going to happen and think out ways of dealing with it. Your body and mind are 'ready for anything' and will function at their best. In other words, tension, even anxiety, in these circumstances is very useful. Normally, during a day our system goes through different phases of tension and relaxation depending on what is happening to us and what we are anticipating. So it is important that, in certain circumstances, we are tense

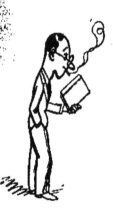

and alert but it is equally important that we are able to relax and 'unwind' in between these periods and it is the inability to do this which leads to problems and to what we normally think of as distressing anxiety.

There are a number of reasons for feeling anxious - fear of physical harm, fear of failure or fear of damage to status ('looking silly' or 'doing the wrong thing') or of damage to a relationship are examples but underlying them all is a 'fear of the unknown', apprehension and uncertainty about what is happening and will happen to you or those close to you. It may be an apparently purposeless feeling which seems quite unrelated to surroundings and circumstances and often the reason it exists relates to happenings many years previously, particularly from childhood and circumstances may now be very different. However, the old feelings and habits persist or have been 'stirred up' again by some traumatic event or current problem.

The level of tension and anxiety in an individual normally fluctuates up and down over a wide range but when a person has been under excessive pressure for long periods of time, this range narrows and they spend much more of their time in a tense and anxious state and are often unable to relax as fully. This becomes more and more uncomfortable as time goes on. It is also increasingly tiring and the physical symptoms of anxiety become more pronounced.

We have already described a number of the signs and symptoms that accompany anxiety but it is useful to have a checklist of the more common of these so that you can recognise them in yourself and begin to accept that what are very real physical symptoms and signs can be caused by 'nerves'. For the body to be at its peak of readiness, it is necessary that:

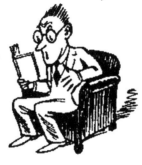

- Muscles are tense and ready for 'fight, flight or fright' and so, because we are 'on edge', we startle easily. Also, the continuing tension leads to;

- Tiredness and weakness and the constant state of alertness makes us irritable and, if it persists for long enough, depressed.

- The tension also causes aches and pains in different parts of the body in a similar way to the way cramp affects us after exercise. It may present as headache, or backache, or pains in the arms or legs or chest, or in any other part of the body.

- So that the muscles can function most efficiently, blood is diverted to them away from organs such as the stomach and remainder of the digestive system and skin, and so;

- Appetite is reduced (although you may, alternatively, 'nibble' more);

- Abdominal discomfort and 'butterflies in the stomach' are felt;

- Diarrhoea may occur because the bowel speeds up and there may be an increased desire to urinate;

- Your hair 'stands on end' and you develop 'goose pimples' and even a 'nervous rash'. Also, to increase the rate at which essential materials, such as oxygen and food, reach the muscles, the heart rate increases and blood pressure rises, causing;

- Palpitations, which really means an awareness of the heart beating and it is usually felt to be going quickly and may even, on occasions, miss a beat.

- The breathing rate also may increase and if it continues 'over breathing' may occur and this may cause;

- Tingling in the fingers and toes because of the changes which occur in some of the chemicals in the blood which affect the nerves and muscles and it may cause;

- Stiffness which can become quite uncomfortable but which is easily reversed.

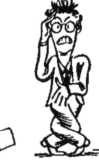

- The breathing may actually stop for a period of seconds or even for a minute or two, basically because there is no need for it, and it stops until the chemicals in the blood have returned to normal. This may give you an uncomfortable awareness, even tightness, around the chest and cause worry that the breathing might not restart; which, however, it always eventually does. Pupils of the eye widen which may cause some;

- Blurring of vision which generally passes off quickly.

All these effects tend to cause some -

- Loss of libido, *ie* loss of sexual interest and, in women, the muscular tension may also make intercourse quite uncomfortable and even painful; in men, there may be impotence and this, in turn, may increase the general state of tension.

- Loss of interest in the activities, hobbies etc that are normally enjoyed. The constant heightened awareness and concentration is eventually counter-productive and we develop;

- Loss of ability to selectively concentrate, *eg* to read a book or magazine and also, because of this, we cannot concentrate on events going on around us and we do not retain them in our mind and so complain of;

- Loss of memory

- Planning and predicting develops into;

- Worry - constantly going over the same situations without coming to any new conclusions and this may contribute to;

- Sleep disturbance

Perhaps, most importantly of all, these changes make you very aware of your body and quite uncertain about it and sensations which you would have probably been unaware of in the past, or just ignored, become very important and worrying. You may even begin to become uncertain about previously strongly-held beliefs about, *eg* religion, or about the future, and this can compound and increase the anxiety.

Anxiety is thought to be an important influence in many 'physical' illnesses, particularly when it persists over a long period of time, *eg* stomach ulcers, ulcerative colitis, high blood pressure, asthma, eczema and arthritis.

Then what??

So, having reached a state of 'nervous exhaustion', fearing for your sanity (which is also quite common as anxiety increases), and afflicted by a multitude of physical symptoms and signs, as outlined above, what do you do? Obviously, you need help, support and reassurance from partners, friends, families and, maybe, doctors or counsellors and this alone may be sufficient to alleviate the anxiety. If there is a particular reason for the anxiety, it may be possible to do something about it and discussion is probably the best way to decide what is wrong and how it can be changed. You may feel that the particular problem is insoluble or a situation unchangeable but there may be some way around it of which you have not thought. It may even involve admitting something to yourself which you have been trying to avoid because it is discomforting and may have implications for changes in the future. Also, change in itself may increase your anxiety and you may stay in the same tense and worrying situation rather than go through the trauma of changing it for something different - however necessary that change may seem.

Nevertheless, even after talking and thinking it through, you may remain quite tense and anxious and, in that situation, it is important that you find ways of relaxing. It may be that listening to a record, chatting with friends, playing a sport or game will help. However, through lack of practice, the ability to relax may become 'rusty' and learning a relaxation exercise (try a tape from the library or chemists) may be useful and this can then be used when tension increases above desired levels.

Medication has often been used for anxiety but if it works, it is usually only helpful short-term. Sometimes antidepressants may help anxiety, whether or not depression is part of the problem

Appendix 3: Depression leaflet

Depression

Depression is very common and can be very distressing.

Common symptoms include:

- Feelings:
  - ◊ Depressed, anxious, angry, confused
- Behaviour:
  - ◊ Isolating, neglectful, erratic, slowed up
  - ◊ Impulsive, argumentative, hostile
- Thoughts:
  - ◊ Content: negative, guilty, non-coping, hopeless, suicidal, paranoid
  - ◊ Types: worrying, confused, forgetful, poor concentration, obsessional, hallucinations
- Physical symptoms
  - ◊ Sleep problems: not getting off, waking in the night and early morning
  - ◊ Appetite: reduced or increased
  - ◊ Fatigue, exhaustion

What can you do about it?

- Accept you are not well & look after yourself —you didn't get depressed deliberately

- There are things that'll help - when you are ready to do them— talk to your mental health worker or family doctor

- Accept help in working out ways to solve them

- Make a list of the problems—it can make them manageable

- If you feel suicidal, tell someone

- Depression gets better– treatment is effective

Index

Note: page numbers in **bold** refer to diagrams, page numbers in *italics* refer to information contained in boxes.

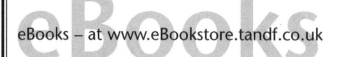